PRAISE FOR *BEYOND ASPIRIN*

"This work on natural cox-2 inl
consumers. As they become educ
enzyme cycloxygenase-2 in hum.
to identify safe and efficacious a
cox-2 inhibitor drugs. Anyone wl
great deal about how to maintain
the onset of some of the most deva ......ases generally associated with aging."

      —Alexander G. Schauss, Ph.D.
> Director, Natural and Medicinal Products Research, Life Sciences Division, AIBMR, Inc., Former, Professor of Natural Products Research, National College of Naturopathic Medicine

"One of the fascinating aspects of herbal medicine is finding of new ways that ancient remedies can help in modern medicine. Recent research outlined in this timely book supports the COX-2 inhibiting properties of many popular herbs, thereby giving them new opportunities for use in modern selfcare and healthcare, and, in turn, giving people safe, lowcost, science-based natural alternatives to potentially toxic conventional drugs."

      —Mark Blumenthal
> Founder and Executive Director, American Botanical Council, Editor, *HerbalGram,* Senior Editor, *The Complete German Commission E Monographs*

"The authors do not refuse the benefits of 'silver-bullet' drugs, but they propose a new insight into traditional herbal medicine. With its perfectly-selected examples of herbal COX-2 inhibitors, the book will stimulate researchers to estimate the value of time-tested herbs. The text supplies a vast list of references, including most recent ones, and can be recommended not only to COX-2 specialists, but also to everyone believing in Nature's harmony."

      — Nina Ivanovska, Ph.D.
> Department of Immunology, Institute of Microbiology, Bulgarian Academy of Sciences

"A brilliant undertaking of a complicated topic. This book makes this knowledge accessible to everyone. People now have a better chance of making the best choices when it comes to their health and the health of their loved ones."

      —Monika Klein, B.H.Ec. C.N.
> Clinical Nutritionist, educator, author and host of the popular television show *Total Health Talk*

"Meticulously researched, intelligently argued, this is a book no one should be without."

      —Jane Buckle, RN. MA. Cert Ed.
> author of *Clinical Aromatherapy in Nursing*

"...a collection of various herbs which contain potential COX-2 inhibiting constituents. The book will be helpful in the search for new materials for further development of new drugs related to COX-2."

      — Shozo Yamamoto, Ph.D.
> Professor Emeritus, Tokushima University, Japan

"In this groundbreaking work, Newmark and Schulick have success-fully combined a knowledge and understanding of the science of to-day and the wisdom of nature to provide us with a glimpse of the medicine of the future."
— **Dr. Greg Kelly, N.D.**
Associate Editor *Alternative Medicine Review*

"A superb treatise on COX-2 inhibition by herbs in relation to dis-eases affecting especially the elderly. I have the opinion that the regu-lar use of herbs as part of the diet would have preventative effects against the debilitating diseases mentioned. This book will serve the common public and inspire those in the medical profession."
—**K.C. Srivastava, Ph.D.**
Associate Professor, Dept. of Environmental Medicine,
Odense University, Denmark

"Science has identified COX-2 inflammation as a major cause of many of our most threatening diseases, and this book offers clear and prac-tical guidance, for patients and physicians, for herbal strategies to control COX-2 inflammation and promote health. As such, it is an important addition to our medical armamentarium. As a practicing surgical physician and an active 'provider' of health care, I am sadly aware that 50% of increased health care costs over the last three years are the result of increasing costs of pharmaceuticals. Not only are modern pharmaceuticals extremely costly, but complications from their use and misuse are the fourth leading cause of death in the United States. In an era where increasing health care costs and patient mor-bidity are ascribed to pharmaceuticals, *Beyond Aspirin* offers timely guidance to doctors and patients seeking intelligent alternatives to synthetic pharmaceuticals."
— **Richard Sarnat, M.D.**
Board-Certified Opthamologist

"*Beyond Aspirin* is a practical and passionate guide for those on the path to wholeness. The research is presented clearly and thoroughly as Newmark and Schulick build a compelling vision for the future use of plants rather than pharmaceutical drugs in the treatment of diseases such as cancer, arthritis and Alzheimer's. This book may be seen as a bridge between science and nature, serving as a model for well-being and life."
—**James Rouse, N.D.**
co-host of Colorado's *Health Time Radio* and
KUSA Colorado's *Optimum Wellness*

"As a chiropractor I am always on the lookout for natural therapies that are efficacious and safe alternatives to dangerous pharmaceuti-cals. This book was both educational and fascinating to read. I rec-ommend it to health care providers and their patients alike."
—**Michael Silbert, D.C.**
Chicago, Illinois

BEYOND ASPIRIN

Nature's Answer
To Arthritis, Cancer
& Alzheimer's Disease

Thomas M. Newmark
and Paul Schulick

HOHM PRESS
2000

Cover design, text layout and design: Shukyo Lin Rainey
Illustrations: Marian Thérèse Newmark

Library of Congress Number: 00-100428
ISBN: 0-934252-82-3

Notice

Beyond Aspirin: Nature's Answer to Arthritis, Cancer, and Alzheimer's Disease is for informational purposes only, and is not a guide for the treatment of any individual's disease or medical condition. The authors hope that the book will provide valuable information about the latest developments in the field of herbal COX-2 inhibition and will stimulate consideration of medical options. Because every person is different, however, a qualifed physician must diagnose conditions and recommend or supervise the use of healing botanicals for the treatment of any health problems. Herbs, other natural remedies, and the information in this book are not substitutes for professional medical care. You should consult a qualified health care practitioner familiar with your medical condition and history before using any of the herbs or recommendations in this book. You should seek the best medical guidance to make your decisions informed and most effective in promoting health.

HOHM PRESS
P.O. Box 2501, Prescott, AZ 86302
800-381-2700
http://www.hohmpress.com
This book was printed in the U.S.A. on acid-free paper using soy ink.

This book is dedicated to our beautiful children,
who have filled our lives with love and purpose.
May their lives be blessed
by the healing power of nature.

ACKNOWLEDGEMENTS

So many people have assisted us in the creation of this book, and we are grateful for their valuable contributions. Within our family, Terry Newmark, the wife of Tom, lovingly drew the botanical illustrations that grace this book, and Paul's son Geremy Schulick had a significant role in researching and preparing the appendix on the traditional uses of the featured herbs. Our dear friends also offered wonderful support. Herb Lewis, who has spent the greater part of his lifetime studying herbs and their medicinal properties, was generous with his insightful suggestions and comments. Shukyo Lin Rainey organized the text and readied it for printing, and she also created the wonderful graphics for the cover. Ruth Austin worked tirelessly to run our farm in Costa Rica and otherwise "tend" to our affairs so we could devote ourselves to this labor of love. Our assistant Jennifer Hart carefully proofed the text, arranged the references, and checked all the many details. To our editors and friends at Hohm Press, we are thankful for your support: it was more than just another book for you, and we are so proud that you shared in our passion for this project. Finally, to the great herbalists and scientists who have preserved the wisdom of healing herbs and advanced the scientific research on their properties, we say only that this work could not have been accomplished without your efforts. It is difficult to single out any one of the teachers and herbalists who has most inspired this work, but we do feel it appropriate to give special thanks to Dr. James A. Duke for his extraordinary scholarship and leadership in our field. To all of the above, we thank you.

CONTENTS

Utnapishtim said to him, to Gilgamesh:
Gilgamesh, you came here;
you strained, you toiled.
What can I give you as you return to your land?
Let me uncover for you, Gilgamesh, a secret thing.
A secret of the gods let me tell you.
There is a plant. Its roots go deep, like the boxthorn;
Its spike will prick your hand like a bramble.
If you get your hands on that plant,
you'll have everlasting life.

The Epic of Gilgamesh, 1600 B.C.E.
(Gardner-Maier Translation)

INTRODUCTION

List making is always a popular diversion, but especially so these days as we transition to the Third Millennium. We find the "One Hundred Greatest Baseball Players of All Time," the "Greatest Inventors of the 20th Century," and so on. But the list that really caught our attention and rather startled us was the one that appeared in the *Wall Street Journal*, October 18, 1999. Just as we were nearing completion of this book, the *Journal* decided to survey the history of preventative medicine. In its full-page review of major current developments, a boxed-off section listed the "past and possible future milestones in preventative medicine."

The first eight achievements, spanning the period from 1796 to 1998, were unquestionably deserving of inclusion on such an exalted listing. First recognizing the 1796 creation of a smallpox vaccine, the *Journal* proceeded to laud Louis Pasteur's discovery of the "germ theory" of disease in 1877; the FDA's approval of Dr. Jonas Salk's polio vaccine in 1955; and the 1964 announcement by the United States Surgeon General that smoking may be a serious health hazard. These and the other milestones cited did indeed alter the medical landscape, changing the way the world looks at disease and its prevention. The *Wall Street Journal* then turned to the future and predicted that in the years 2002-2003 "COX-2 inhibitors likely to prove successful in preventing colon cancer in high-risk patients."

COX-2 inhibitors refer to compounds, both synthetic and natural, that have the ability to inhibit an enzyme in the body referred to as cyclooxygenase-2. It is likely that you have already heard of COX-2 inhibitors. Significant advertising has accompanied the release of the first pharmaceutical to have that effect. If you have not yet heard of COX-2, then we assure you that by the end of your reading of this book you will know all you need to know about how to tame this potentially inflammatory beast.

When it acknowledged that COX-2 inhibition would earn a place on the list of the most important preventative medical accomplishments of all time, the *Wall Street Journal* was focusing on the prevention of colon cancer. Frankly, the inhibition of COX-2 is even more remarkable than the *Journal's* high praise would indicate, for the prevention of colon cancer is just the beginning of what will be accomplished with this medical revolution. A growing body of science is demonstrating that COX-2 inhibition prevents or reverses a number of currently life-threatening cancers.

Indeed, on January 18, 2000 the *New York Times*, in its lead article in the "Science Times," noted that "two decades of accumulating research 'support' the idea that blocking the cox-2 enzyme might prevent cancer." In addition to preventing colon cancer, the *New York Times* observed that fifty studies "show that blocking cox-2 can prevent premalignant and malignant tumors in animals, and not just colon cancers. The drugs appear effective for bladder, skin, and esophageal cancers as well."

The story of COX-2 inhibition is both as new as the October *Wall Street Journal* article and as old as Hippocrates. It is true that pharmaceutical companies are rushing to develop and market synthetic COX-2 inhibitors, such as Celebrex® and Vioxx®. It is also true, however, that thousands of years ago Hippocrates was prescribing an herbal COX-2 inhibitor for pain and inflammation. As is so often the case, the pharmaceutical industry attempts to synthetically recreate the extraordinary healing properties of traditional herbal medicine. While there *can* be a time and a place for synthetic COX-2 inhibitors, there is *always* wisdom in integrating the safe and traditional herbal COX-2 inhibitors that have proven to be profoundly effective over thousands of years.

As this book will carefully explain, COX-2 inflammation lies at the root of many diseases, including cancer, Alzheimer's disease and many forms of arthritis. Those diseases are often expressions of a mind and body struggling and succumbing to the fires of out-of-control COX-2 inflammation. As this book will explain, the pharmaceutical COX-2 inhibitors are uncertain in both the scope of their inhibitory powers and the nature of their side effects. It is precisely for these reasons that a time-tested herbal program to inhibit COX-2 inflammation is central to the medical efforts to reverse those disease processes.

We are fortunate that the biochemical sciences are now able to identify the specific herbs and their constituents that inhibit the COX-2 inflammation process. Drawing upon the collective wisdom of traditional medical systems and modern science, this book identifies the revered herbs from around the world that most powerfully and comprehensively inhibit COX-2 inflammation and reverse the disease processes born of that inflammation. That is the promise, the medical revolution, of COX-2 herbal inhibition.

CHAPTER ONE

Arthritis—From NSAIDS to the "Safe Aspirin"

Arthritis touches the lives of millions around the world. It is a painful, pervasive and disabling touch. In the U.S. alone, it is estimated that approximately forty million people suffer from osteoarthritis (OA), more currently being called osteoarthrosis, with an additional two to three million suffering from rheumatoid arthritis (RA). These are but two of over one hundred conditions comprehended within the term "arthritis." Modern health professionals have struggled to deliver safe relief from the often chronic pain associated with these diseases, but for decades the pain intervention of choice has been the long-term use of potentially dangerous nonsteroidal anti-inflammatory drugs (NSAIDS) like aspirin, ibuprofen and naproxen. Unfortunately, such long-term medication carries with it risks of serious side effects such as kidney damage, peptic ulcers and associated severe hemorrhaging and perforation.

As the use of NSAIDS persists, and as the users age, the risks of serious toxicities increase. Elderly patients on NSAIDS experience a much higher rate of complication for ulcers, gastrointestinal irritation and kidney failure than the overall population. In elderly patients, as many as 6% to 9% of NSAID users will require hospitalization due to serious gastrointestinal toxicity. Like many elderly, patients with rheumatoid arthritis already have compromised physiologies, and one large database analysis indicated that their chronic use of NSAIDS increased their risk of GI-related hospitalizations and death sixfold and twofold, respectively.

A study published in 1998 in the *American Journal of Medicine* reported that an estimated 107,000 people are admitted each year to hospitals as a result of complications due to the use of NSAIDS. It is estimated that as many as 16,500 people died last year from serious complications from NSAID-induced bleeding. To put that number in perspective, it is almost identical to the number of people whose deaths last year were attributed to AIDS-related conditions.

THE "SAFE ASPIRIN" ARRIVES

In December 1998 the U.S. Food and Drug Administration (FDA) approved a drug called Celebrex (celecoxib) for the treatment of both osteoarthritis and rheumatoid arthritis. This announcement was welcomed by the popular press as the long-awaited invention of a "safe aspirin." The medical community was optimistic about Celebrex being a revolutionary advance in arthritis pain relief, and Wall Street hailed the drug as the next Viagra®, with potential annual sales estimated to be in the $5 billion range. There have been reports that in the first eleven months of Celebrex's introduction, over twelve million prescriptions for the drug were written, and it is anticipated that there will be eighteen million prescriptions written in the year 2000. In the first nine months following licensing, Celebrex generated over $1 billion in sales. During the period May-October, 1999, approximately 2.2 million prescriptions were written for Vioxx, Merck's COX-2 inhibitor, FDA-approved for arthritis and menstrual pain. It is estimated that literally tens of millions of people will take Celebrex, Vioxx, or related compounds for pain relief in lieu of taking traditional NSAIDS-like aspirin. To put the anticipated use of these new drugs in perspective, in 1995 alone there were thirty-five million prescriptions written for NSAIDS, and billions of dollars more were spent on non-prescription

3

lower-dosage over-the-counter NSAIDS. Over the course of the "Aspirin Century," from the introduction of aspirin nearly one hundred years ago, it is estimated that over one trillion aspirin doses have been taken. It is fair to say that every person who has ever taken an aspirin or a traditional NSAID is a prime candidate for "the revolution of COX-2 inhibitors."

Although clinical results are obviously preliminary, and many of the early studies have yet to be published, it is appropriate to acknowledge that Celebrex and Vioxx appear to offer relief from pain and inflammation that is similar to traditional NSAIDS (about a 70% efficacy rate), with a decreased incidence of the unwelcome side effects associated with those NSAIDS. For example, a recent University of Chicago study of over five thousand patients with arthritis reported that with Celebrex there was an "absolute" and "unequivocal" significant reduction of "gastrointestinal events" compared to traditional NSAIDS.

CHAPTER TWO

Understanding Inflammation and Balance

The over one hundred manifestations of arthritis share a common denominator: pain. And this pain is often caused or exacerbated by inflammation. The medical meaning of the term "inflammation" is extremely simple—the affected part of the body, or the entire body, becomes inflamed. There is swelling; the affected areas or the entire body get hot; white blood cells begin to wage serious battle; often there is pain. Everyone has experienced inflammation; just think of all the times you have had some form of "itis"—like tonsillitis or dermatitis.

Many people are, sadly, intimately familiar with another "itis," namely, arthritis. Arthritis literally means, and is often defined as, an inflammation of the joints in the body. Contrary to commonly held belief, it is not an inevitable condition of aging. It is a disease condition in

5

which joints and their connective tissue degenerate; joints, cartilage and bone become tender and painful; and there is often some degree of inflammation.

There is a trend in the medical and scientific communities to rename the most common form of arthritis "osteoarthrosis," to reflect the present belief that osteoarthritis is more an expression of cartilage and joint deterioration than inflammation. While we acknowledge that inflammatory processes do not necessarily dominate in cases of osteoarthritis, underlying inflammatory processes or associated conditions—like free-radical stress and pain-receptor sensitization—often significantly aggravate the osteoarthritis condition. Moreover, it is unquestionable that inflammatory processes stimulate bone deterioration and can impede bone and cartilage repair. Accordingly, while we acknowledge that osteoarthritis does not always carry associated inflammation with it, we believe that there is a powerful interconnection between inflammatory processes and the progress of osteoarthritis.

Here is how the most common form of arthritis, osteoarthritis, arises: There is protective cartilage in the joints, and this cartilage is a soft and flexible tissue that helps hold the bones in place, and gives our joints both strength and flexibility. This protective cartilage is constantly being dismantled, repaired and replaced. Just like other tissues

6

in the body, the protective cartilage at some point becomes damaged, exhausted, or just loses its elasticity. It can be likened to a rubber band that gets old, starts to lose its ability to stretch and snap back, and then gets brittle. If the cartilage weakens in that manner, it has lost its usefulness and the body wants to replace it. That's when the body's salvage team moves into the picture. Its job is to dismantle and recycle the cartilage that has entered the winter of its life. As the old, worn out cartilage is salvaged, it is imperative that the body creates an equal amount of new cartilage to replace the old tissue. There is supposed to be, therefore, a perfect balance between the salvage and re-creation of cartilage. If the body does not create enough new cartilage to take the place of the old, the bones lose their soft protection, resulting in weakness, pain and loss of flexibility.

A notion of a perfect balance between cartilage dismantling and cartilage recreation is somewhat idealized. What really happens is that things start out that way, but as we age the process begins to wobble like a tired gyroscope. The repair processes go on, however, as though it's business as usual, but these processes aren't what they used to be. It's like a pitcher who has a 95-m.p.h. fastball when he's twenty-five, but at twenty-eight has lost maybe a mile or two. At first, no one really notices, but then a point is reached when he can't get the hitters out any more. It's a colorful analogy, and it's

7

basically descriptive of the repair process for most of us. As we age we are still in the cartilage repair game (we still go through the motions), but the process is simply not quite up to our youthful standards. That's okay for a while, for most of us will be functioning near enough to effective balance that we can still operate as we've been used to. Maybe we will be a bit stiff after exercise or hiking, but we can work the joints, the cartilage will loosen up, and we will get by.

With the passage of time, with each fresh pound of weight, and with the consumption of foods that are not ideal, the repair mechanisms begin to lag. The tears and nicks in the cartilage can become inflamed; and, ironically, the inflammation process, which in itself is natural, creates chemicals that accelerate the breaking down of cartilage. The tired gyroscope really starts to wobble, and what had been a problem of degrees has become a major problem of kind. The stiff joint that hadn't quite worked deteriorates into a joint that becomes locked, grossly inflamed and doesn't work at all. There is this bizarre irony: inflammation is present to marshal the body's repair and protection mechanism, but with the accelerating inflammation, the cartilage starts to literally fall apart. The inflammation of the joint, which began in response to injury and was designed to help restore balance, becomes our own worst enemy. In a fundamental way, **the disease condition of certain forms**

of arthritis are a result of too much inflammation, and osteoarthritis becomes exacerbated by inflammatory and associated processes.

At this juncture it is important to note that not all inflammation is bad. To the contrary, fevers are a part of the healing process; so, too, is pain. You have certainly heard the expression that pain is nature's way of telling us that something is wrong. That is absolutely correct. At the point of inflammation, at the point where bone abrades bone, there is an urgent need for the body to signal distress. To use a crude but descriptive analogy, a mechanic cannot repair your car when it is barreling down the highway; for repair to occur, the car must be brought to rest. Our common sense tells us that our body's repair mechanisms function in a similar manner. If there is damage to our joints and tissues, therefore, we need to bring them to a state of rest. Just think of how doctors put broken bones in a cast to keep them from moving. But, how do we know when to stop moving the damaged joint so that our healing forces can be best brought to bear? How does our body even know when a joint is damaged at all?

You know the answer: when pain leaps from cell to cell, alerting the entire body that the damaged area requires special attention. For instance, you stub your toe and it seems that almost immediately every cell in your body is on alert and aware of the pain, aware of the need to stop stubbing your toe. Or, your bones, perhaps in your knee or wrist, begin to rub together, and every cell is again alerted by pain that damage is occurring and that the joint must get repaired.

So, our quarrel is not with inflammation, but with excessive inflammation. In an osteoarthritic joint, certain inflammatory chemicals are produced in an excessive amount which, as we explained, over-stimulate cartilage destruction. The chemicals that stimulate this imbalanced destruction are by-products of a particular enzyme in the body called **cycloxygenase-2 (COX-2)**. In other words, joint tissues in the body generally exist in a state of working equilibrium—between tissue degradation and tissue recreation—until the by-products of an overstimulated COX-2 enzyme can create a condition of inflammation that destroys the balance.

Does this process sound a little complex? Consider a hillside with a gentle slope. Imagine that the soil on the hillside is deep, moist and rich, and more than ample to cover the hard rock below. In that rich soil grow grasses and flowers, watered from time to time by gentle rains. With each rain, only a little topsoil is lost, because the plant roots secure the soil. And as the plants die over time, they decompose and form new topsoil, and the balance between gentle rain, topsoil loss and topsoil restoration is maintained. But think about what happens if a machine or wheel cuts a track on the hillside. The plants in that one location are damaged, and with the next rain a slight increase in normal erosion takes place. The roots of the plants no longer secure the soil and soon a gully forms. When the rains come again, more topsoil is lost, the gully grows deeper, and there is less organic matter to recycle into new topsoil. The balance of the ecology has been damaged. If the imbalance is severe enough, or continues over a long enough period of time, the raw rock of the hillside can become exposed.

The ecology of the hillside, like the ecology of the human elbow joint, for example, is all a question of balance. If the protective tissue, the soil of the body, is degraded too rapidly, then the "hard rock" of the joint can become exposed. This may sound too simple now, but that's all there is to our physiology—a question of balance.

Approximately one-third of people over age thirty-five show a degree of the cartilage deterioration that characterizes osteoarthritis—that characterizes "joint imbalance." The reason why this joint imbalance arises more frequently as people age is also fairly easy to understand. For instance, when a child cuts his finger, the skin heals quickly and strongly. When we age, the healing often takes longer and may not be as complete. In general, when we are younger we can create new tissue more quickly and heal wounds more effectively, and this translates directly to cartilage tissue in the joints. If there is some imbalance (which is always present to some

11

extent) in the cartilage tissue when we are young, we can fix it quickly and completely. But, as we age, our general decline in wound-healing ability makes us less able to respond to joint imbalances as they arise. We seem to lose a step in responding to these tiny imbalances that inevitably build up. A momentum of imbalance begins to develop, as each increment of imbalance creates a little more inflammation, which triggers a little more tissue deterioration, and which leaves us increasingly behind the tissue re-creation process. Picture this process like this: You drop two steel balls at precisely the same time, one in air and one in molasses. The ball that drops in air continues to accelerate as it falls. Oddly enough, the ball dropped in molasses is also accelerating, but at a much slower rate. With each passing moment, as both balls are dropping and accelerating, the ball dropped in air is greatly outdistancing the one dropped in molasses. The ball in molasses could be said to be losing ground. The analogy to aging is precise. The disintegration of tissue (the ball dropping in air) is accelerating extremely quickly in conditions of inflammation. Even though the re-creation of tissue (ball in molasses) is also accelerating and trying to keep up, it keeps falling farther and farther behind. Therefore, because wound healing as we age is moving as though through molasses compared to the rapid state of tissue destruction, we simply can't restore balance. As a result, the cartilage tissue simply breaks down.

The flip side of this process is how we deal with inflammation, which is the core concept of this book and therefore essential to understand. Not only do we lose the ability to quickly regenerate new tissue as we age, but we are also losing a step in resisting and maintaining balance in the inflammation process. The flu or cold that only momentarily disrupts our activity when we are young can throw a weaker, older physiology into a tailspin. Due to the accumulated wear and tear on the body, its ability to keep inflammation in check is somewhat diminished as it ages. If inflammation persists too long, or heats up too much, then the chemicals created in that state of chronic inflammation trigger increased deterioration of joint tissue.

The situation just described is a double whammy. Not only does an aging physiology lose a step in regenerating tissue, it also loses a step in taming the fires of inflammation that literally "burn" the old tissue. The key here is the absence of balance. As we've noted, inflammation in itself is not a bad thing; the activity of the COX-2 enzyme in creating inflammation is a normal, natural part of the body responding to stress and challenge. However, when the COX-2 inflammatory process is aggravated and over-stimulates cartilage deterioration, the problem of arthritis can become exacerbated.

This description of the arthritis disease process points the way to the two things we must do to help restore balance in the diseased joint. First, we need to provide the aging body with stronger tools for controlling the fires of inflammation and for promoting wound healing. These tools are the herbal COX-2 inhibitors, which will be our focus throughout this book. Second, we need to adopt a more unbounded approach to healing—one that includes acting more in alignment with nature's impulses. We will discuss this second issue in the last chapter of this book. Doing one without the other is incomplete—to respond effectively to a state of excessive inflammation we must address both.

In our times, imbalance reigns. Joints are inflamed, cartilage is in shreds, and over forty million people in the United States alone suffer from osteoarthritis. Definitive evidence affirms that more than 70% of the elderly suffer from some osteoarthritis of the knee joint. The problem of osteoarthritis is one that touches virtually every family.

Everything said about osteoarthritis can be multiplied for rheumatoid arthritis (RA), which affects fewer individuals (perhaps only one in one hundred), but is often far more disabling. Rheumatoid arthritis is more a disease of the young, versus the older profile of the osteoarthritis sufferer. Three times more women have rheumatoid arthritis than do men, and most sufferers are between thirty-five and fifty years of age. The dominant distinguishing symptom of rheumatoid arthritis is *generalized* inflammation. The rheumatoid arthritis inflammation may, of course, be confined to just the cartilage in joints, but rheumatoid arthritis can also affect the entire body, causing such varied symptoms as loss of appetite, loss of energy and a powerful sense of simply being "unwell." For some, rheumatoid arthritis can result in serious joint deformity and immobility. The fundamental condition of rheumatoid arthritis is inflammation, and once again an over-stimulated COX-2 enzyme lies at the core of the problem.

Thus far, we have learned that cartilage comes and goes, but that the maintenance of cartilage balance basically works until the inflammation process, as we have broadly defined it, accelerates the disintegration of the tissue. It is a classic case of being hoisted on one's own petard, especially when you understand that a petard is an explosive device, which is one way to look at the inflammatory chemicals created at the site of inflammation. When inflammation and its associated processes go haywire, the bones lose their protective tissue, bone can rub against bone, joints can lock up, and what was once a manageable stream of inflammatory chemicals can become an out-and-out Class-V whitewater disaster. Typically, when the joints become heated and swollen, people have taken aspirin. One hundred years of aspirin, one trillion pills. They took aspirin for one absolutely valid reason: the drug worked to relieve or at least reduce inflammation, and to restore the ability to function more manageably in life.

This introduction to the term COX-2 cannot be fully appreciated without a brief lesson on why aspirin works. From the introduction of aspirin at the turn of the twentieth century, and for the next eighty years or so, no one had any idea why aspirin relieved pain. Then, Sir John Vane discovered that aspirin decreased the production of inflammatory hormones, or chemicals, called prostaglandins. Prostaglandins were known to be created by the cyclooxygenase enzyme. This was key. Once we knew that aspirin reduced inflammatory prostaglandins, we could begin to solve the inflammation puzzle.

The aspirin mystery was at least partially solved. If a person was suffering from an excess of inflammation, such as with arthritis, then taking a substance that inhibited the creation of the inflammatory prostaglandin was just what the doctor ordered, literally. Aspirin was a doctor's best friend. Inhibiting cyclooxygenase inhibited the creation of inflammatory prostaglandins—no ifs, ands or buts. Therefore, many millions of arthritis sufferers, together with those suffering other inflammations, guzzled aspirins as fast as possible. There was a problem, however. All too often the chronic use of NSAIDS caused severe bleeding and kidney damage—even death. **These dire consequences arose because NSAIDS, some worse than others, disrupted the formation of inflammatory**

prostaglandins, but also inhibited the balancing and protective features of the COX enzyme. It turned out that COX, or one still yet-to-be discovered enzymatic expression of it, was essential for proper kidney function and for protecting the stomach. If you chronically inhibited all COX activity, such as with long-term use of NSAIDS for pain relief, you risked damaging critical organ systems in the body. Of course, this was frustrating to both patients and conventional doctors. People in arthritic pain or discomfort were desperate for relief, but the medical risk was often too high to allow them to take NSAIDS on a chronic basis.

THE DISCOVERY OF COX-2

In 1991, scientists led by Dr. Philip Needleman made a crucial discovery: the COX enzyme was not one enzyme, it was actually two. Both COX enzymes had the ability to metabolize, or burn, a particular fat in the body. The enzyme that came to be known as COX-1, however, was the one responsible for maintaining housekeeping balance—scientists called it homeostasis—in our kidneys and stomach. The other expression of COX, not surprisingly an isoenzyme called COX-2, was identified as the one responsible for the creation of inflammatory prostaglandins out of the fat called arachidonic acid.

In the ensuing years, researchers raced to locate a "silver bullet" that would disrupt the inflammatory COX-2 pathway without unduly inhibiting the protective, housekeeping features of COX-1. This research located numerous COX-2 inhibitors, some of which selectively inhibited COX-2. What this means is that the inhibitor had a particular appetite, or preference, for interfering with the COX-2 enzyme. Conversely, because it preferred the COX-2 enzyme, it tended to leave the beneficial features of the COX-1 enzyme alone. Scientists at Monsanto located a highly specific COX-2 inhibitor called celecoxib, known commonly as Celebrex. This specialty compound had 375 to 400 times more affinity for COX-2 than COX-1. In simple terms, in theory, it blocked the creation of the inflammatory hormones hundreds of times more powerfully than it disrupted processes in the kidney and stomach. To understand this concept of selective inhibition, we want you to imagine a big back-yard party, with eight hundred glasses of flavored milk—four hundred each of chocolate and vanilla—set out for the guests. Imagine, further, that an icy wind sweeps over the area in which the party is taking place—a wind so intelligent that it can seek out only the chocolate-flavored milk. If this intelligent, freezing wind had the same selective ability of Celebrex, then when it froze all four hundred glasses of chocolate milk, it would end up freezing perhaps only one or two glasses of vanilla.

Another selective COX-2 inhibitor, a Merck synthesized compound called Vioxx, appears to have a thousand times greater preference for inhibiting COX-2 (freezing the chocolate milk) over inhibiting COX-1 (not freezing the vanilla milk). In other words, you could give a patient enough of this drug to significantly inhibit the COX-2 enzyme, while its effects on COX-1 would theoretically be kept to a minimum. Many other pharmaceutical "silver bullets" are in development. But, the FDA's late-1998 approval of Celebrex as the first COX-2 inhibiting drug is a recognition that it showed substantial promise as a NSAID that could often reduce pain and inflammation without inducing the magnitude or frequency of severe side effects common to other NSAIDS.

As stated above, the pain relief efficacy rate for Celebrex has been clinically measured at approximately 70%. In an early test on Celebrex use for post-operative pain, the data suggest that Celebrex was as effective as conventional narcotics. Celebrex has also been shown to be as effective as Naproxen in relieving osteoarthritic hip pain. Researchers associated with Merck, the creator of Vioxx, report that Vioxx relieves pain associated with menstrual cramps, and the FDA has now approved the use of Vioxx for the treatment of menstrual pain. Hence the exalted status of these drugs as the pharmaceutical industry's first "safe aspirins."

CHAPTER THREE

COX-2 Extends
To the World of Cancer

In Chapter Two we began to explore the relationship between arthritis and the damage to the cartilage from excessive COX-2 inflammation. We now understand— based on a century-long experience of controlling arthritis inflammation with aspirin and on the groundbreaking work of Sir John Vane—that arthritis is born of COX-2 inflammation, and that inhibiting COX-2 offers arthritis relief.

The most fascinating aspect of the inflammation connection to arthritis is that, while inflammation is a natural response to injury and an important part of the body's strategy to repair damage, when inflammation is too great it can result in even worse cartilage damage. This is a picture of damage by friendly fire, where the body's fighting forces gets overzealous, the bullets begin to fly off in uncontrolled directions, and the defended cartilage is actually a victim of the rescue efforts. The key, as always, is balance: where breaking down the cartilage is balanced with re-creation of tissue, we are fine. Where the wrecking efforts are excessive, or conversely where our wound-healing and repair abilities are impaired, we see accelerated and cellular mutation and tissue deterioration.

This issue of damage by friendly fire carries over to other disease conditions, such as cancers and Alzheimer's disease. Alzheimer's will be considered at length toward the end of this book, but we turn our attention now to the mechanisms by which imbalanced inflammation contributes to the growth of cancers in various organs.

It is crucial to note that we have not seen any relationship between the manifestation of COX-2 inflammation into arthritis and a manifestation of COX-2 inflammation into cancer—one does not seem to lead or relate to the other. The relationship is between the over-expression of COX-2 inflammation in organs and the existence of cancers in those body systems. What we are discovering is that inflammation is a condition underlying both of these disease expressions. To make this point clear, imagine a balloon that is being squeezed. The balloon will bulge in different ways depending on the angle of the pressure and the weaknesses in the balloon. In the same way, pressure on the body coming from

22

excessive COX-2 inflammation can cause the body to bulge (or break) in different ways. Depending upon where that inflammation arises, as it relates to the strength and weaknesses of the particular body, different diseases can occur. We emphasize this point to make sure that you do not conclude that having one disease will lead to the other—they share common "breeding grounds," but they are separate expressions. A scientific understanding of this relationship is just now dawning. Let's look at the patterns that are emerging.

Scientists have observed what had been an unexplained relationship between long-term use of NSAIDS for arthritis pain relief and a *lower* incidence of colon cancer. In 1999, the German Cancer Research Center reported that prostaglandin inhibitors such as NSAIDS "have been shown to halve the incidence of colorectal cancer in man." The Department of Medicine of a major U.S. hospital reported in 1998 that colorectal cancer "is the third leading cause of cancer-related mortality and a significant public health problem in the United States. Aspirin and other nonsteroidal anti-inflammatory drugs reduced the incidence of colorectal cancers and related mortality by 30% to 60%." Whether the percentage reduction is thirty, fifty or sixty percent, that is obviously a profound reduction of colon cancer. Frankly, at first blush it is a confounding relationship, for long-term NSAID use is clearly stressful on the physiology, often inducing ulcers and serious bleeding, and sometimes causing side effects so profound as to lead to thousands of deaths per year. Yet, those same drugs, which were designed merely to reduce pain, have been observed worldwide to significantly reduce the incidence of colon cancer. On a side note, even though this relationship has long been observed, doctors have been reluctant to prescribe chronic NSAID use as a chemopreventative for colon cancer for one simple reason: long-term use of such drugs is plainly dangerous, and the available evidence on colon cancer chemoprevention was not sufficiently powerful to overcome the incontrovertible health risks associated with NSAID use.

As another element in the emerging relationship between COX-2 expression and cancer, the COX-2 enzyme metabolizes or burns a specific type of fat called arachidonic acid. Scientists discovered in 1999 that when arachidonic acid is metabolized by a cousin enzyme called 5-lipoxygenase, the by-product of that metabolism actually feeds cancer cells of the prostate. Although this is not a direct COX-2 metabolic issue, the relationship between 5-lipoxygenase and prostate cancer confirms that the oxidation of arachidonic acid can be a primary fuel for cancer growth.

We also know that COX-2 is normally not significantly present or expressed in certain healthy organ tissue, like that found in a healthy pancreas. Researchers discovered, however, that COX-2 is sixty times more prevalent in a cancerous pancreas than in one not exhibiting cancer. A recent study published on October 6, 1999 in the *Journal of the American Medical Association* was particularly compelling. Researchers at the Royal College of Surgeons in Ireland showed the powerful relationship between COX-2 and cancer. Doctors performed biopsies on colon tissue from seventy-six patients with colorectal cancer and from fourteen individuals without cancer. All seventy-six cancer tumors showed the expression of COX-2, while none of the colon tissue from non-cancer patients reflected COX-2 expression. The researchers further found that the more advanced the tumor, the more likely that the tumor would express high levels of COX-2. Researchers also established a strong negative correlation between COX-2 expression and five-year survival likelihood. The lead doctor on the research team noted that the role of COX-2 in cancer remains unclear, but that "COX-2 has been found in other . . . cancers such as gastric and esophagus . . . breast, ovary, skin, bladder and lung. . . ." The next month, scientists in Sweden published in a leading research journal called *Gut* their research indicating that elevated COX-2 levels were present in eighteen of twenty patients with primary adenocarcinomas located in the rectum. Scientists had never even heard of COX-2 until the early 1980s, and most of the public at large had not heard of it until 1999. Now we know that it is a factor in many of our most threatening diseases.

CHAPTER FOUR

The Intimacies Between COX-2 and Cancer

The relationship between the activity of COX-2 and cancer is emerging. As COX-2 activity increases, cancers increase. Conversely, as the activity of COX-2 is inhibited, colon and other cancers appear to diminish in frequency. Why? What does an over-expression of COX-2 do? What compound or condition does it create to cause cancer cells to grow, spread and succeed in the body? It turns out that cancer cells, like other living organisms and tissues, are on a mission to live and proliferate. They evolve strategies for survival and for spreading—for metastasizing—throughout the body. We are coming to understand that cancer cells use inflammation, born of COX-2, as a mechanism for survival and growth.

The precise ways that inflammation itself supports cancer are not fully explored, but we are beginning to recognize a biological model that has the following elements:

Fuel

Cancer cells grow rapidly and need high-octane fuel for their growth. As we have previously explained, many cancer cells thrive on fuels that are made from a fat in the body called arachidonic acid. You may recall that in 1999 scientists discovered that one of these fuels is responsible for the growth of prostate cancer. The importance of this "high octane fuel source" for cancer cell growth cannot be overstated. For example, prostate cancer cells are difficult to eradicate—they prove resistant to many forms of irradiation and chemotherapy. Scientists from the University of Virginia Cancer Center published their findings (in the U.S. Government's *Proceedings of the National Academy of Sciences*) that if prostate cancer cells are deprived of their fuel, then within one to two hours the prostate cancer cells begin a massive and rapid mass suicide. This mass suicide, referred to as "apoptosis," is described in more detail below.

Stickiness

Cancer cells are dedicated to finding new places to reside in the body. They would not be the only cells that are totally focused on such a mission. Indeed, we could intelligently argue that all cells are programmed, and have as their goal, reproduction and proliferation. Sperm cells swim furiously and battle impossible odds to fuse with the egg. The cells of a fertilized egg differentiate, multiply and create organ systems in a fortnight. What is true for the individual cell is true for that unique collection of cells we call a living organism. Monarch butterflies migrate thousands of miles to nest and breed, and we know how salmon will fight to inevitable death to return to the place (how could they possibly remember which one?) where they were spawned, to spawn again. This is the way of life, and the DNA or cosmic plan immanent within cellular, plant and animal life will passionately pursue reproduction and proliferation.

A cancer cell, stuck somewhere inside some organ culvert, isolated from the currents of life coursing within the body, and surrounded by "hostile" DNA that views it as an enemy to be destroyed . . . how does it break free? How does it loose itself from its microscopic lump in some nook of the body (where, if it remains confined, it is not likely to cause much damage, much less death), and get the free range that it desires? After all, people typically do not die from having cancer, they die from the *spread* of cancer. One of cancer's best strategies for proliferation involves platelets. Platelets are circulating throughout the body; think of them as sticky surfboards. If a cancer cell can stick onto a blood platelet, it will be carried by that platelet to another site of potential growth in the body.

And so on, and so on. The more sticky surfboard surfaces, the better. With inflammation we normally see an increase of blood flow and platelets in the inflamed region, and thus an increase in sticky surfboard platelets swirling around or near cancer cells. Blood, our best friend, the very current of life within our bodies, filled with platelets that perform absolutely indispensable functions, this very stuff of life is sometimes co-opted by malignant cells and used to hasten our death. Remember: it's all in the balance of these forces.

The stickiness factor in cancer proliferation is commanding increased scientific attention. It is known, for example, that cigarette smoking and stress result in higher platelet aggregation factors. Although the association between cancer and these lifestyle factors has been documented for decades, the associated increase in platelet stickiness is often ignored when discussing the whys of cancer. More diabolical is the ability of cancer cells to make platelets even stickier than they normally are so they may fulfill their frantic mission to survive and dominate.

Angiogenesis

One of the hormones made by COX-2 (and not COX-1) from the specific body fat called arachidonic acid is a blood vessel growth stimulator named "thromboxane." The body stimulates the production of thromboxane, for example, when there is traumatized or damaged tissue, for if tissue is damaged we need to grow new tissue, and that new tissue needs oxygen and food. Hence the body's wisdom of stimulating new blood vessels. If the body is chronically inflamed, the rush of this hormone called thromboxane stimulates the growth of new blood vessels into regions that may contain cancer tumors. This process of stimulating new blood vessel growth is called "angiogenesis." These new blood vessels allow the tumor to receive fuel (food and oxygen) and offer the additional cancer-promoting feature of bringing to the tumor more "sticky surfboard" platelets as potential carriers of cancer cells. We will later explain the significance of thromboxane being stimulated by COX-2 and not COX-1.

Cellular Proliferation

As we have seen, when COX-2 catalyzes or reacts with arachidonic acid, one of the byproducts is a prostaglandin that accelerates cellular growth (proliferation). This makes sense. If there is damage to the body and tissue is wounded, it would be natural and beneficial for the body to try to heal the wound as promptly as possible. One way to heal a wound is to stimulate cells to reproduce more aggressively so that repair can be accomplished more quickly. It is thus a healthy strategy to have an inflammatory prostaglandin promote cellular reproduction—but that can get out of balance. If there is a malignancy in the body (and there often is somewhere), then chemicals that promote cellular proliferation can have the unintended effect of promoting the growth of the tumor cells. Again, it is a question of balance, but the point is that promoting cell growth, a normal part of the COX-2 inflammation response, also promotes tumor growth. And, if an area of the body is constantly inflamed, the obvious effect is the constant overstimulation of cancer cell proliferation.

Bad Cells Refuse to Die

COX-2 metabolites have the effect of inhibiting something called apoptosis. That is the medical term for programmed cell death, which is literally cellular suicide. Sometimes, old or diseased cells *should* kill themselves—the body wants to clear the underbrush and promote the growth of new, healthy cells. It is part of the cell's life cycle that at some point it should turn itself off and die. But what if there is damage or injury to part of the body? In such a case, it might be smart to conserve the old cells because other cells have already been lost to some trauma or injury. This is precisely what happens during inflammation—the body thinks that it needs every cell to heal the wound, and it therefore creates substances that can turn off the suicide switch in the body. This is great for the healthy cells, but it's a bad thing for malignant cells that would otherwise be programmed to self-destruct. One of the ways the body turns off the suicide switch is through expressing COX-2. There is strong evidence that the over-expression of COX-2 and inflammatory prostaglandins results in the unfortunate inhibition of cancer cell apoptosis.

Chaos

When a cut gets infected, we notice that it gets a little puffy and warm to the touch. This is modest inflammation, and it is normal. If the inflammation is a little worse, as with a severe sprain, the inflamed area can become extremely swollen, tender and hot. If an area gets profoundly inflamed, as with rheumatoid arthritis, the tissues lose their normal shape and form, and deterioration occurs to the point where the tissue becomes severely deformed and dysfunctional. Although the levels or seriousness of inflammation can vary widely, from a cut to rheumatoid arthritis, wherever there is inflammation there is typically some warmth, swelling and redness. What is happening to cause this?

When a tissue is injured (as from infection or trauma), it releases chemical signals that are like a summons for help. These chemical signals go by many exotic names, like cytokines and chemokines, but their role is to recruit certain other cells into the damaged area. The recruited cells come in many forms and also have exotic names, but mainly, they are different kinds of white blood cells rushing to the rescue. This leads to the swelling of inflammation.

Picture an inflamed area engorged with angry white blood cells, firing away with their oxidative ray guns. That's right, these biological cavalrymen shoot bursts of free radicals of oxygen at invaders. We mean this literally—that's one of the ways white blood cells work. They work by producing free radicals to act as biological thieves, to steal electrons to assist the breakdown of damaged tissue or invading/foreign substances. It is great to destabilize the cells we need to kill or remove, but destabilizing lots of surrounding healthy cells can obviously have serious consequences, potentially leading to DNA mutation and cancer cell growth.

Among the free radicals that can arise at points of inflammation is a special and little understood molecule called nitric oxide. Scientists have just discovered this molecule, and it appears to play a role in helping an inflamed area's cry for help travel through the body. Although we don't know all that much about the workings of nitric oxide, we do know that it is goes in and out of existence very rapidly, is concentrated in inflamed areas, and is thought to play a role in the formation of many diseases, particularly cancers. It also is created by Viagra, which is another story altogether. The scientists who recently discovered this molecule were awarded a Nobel Prize for their efforts. Someone else will likely win another Nobel Prize for determining the precise function of this ephemeral biochemical.

In addition, as white blood cells rush into the inflamed area, the tissues in that area begin to break down, discrete areas in the body begin to lose integrity, and the bright lines that once separated one tissue from another get blurred in the puree of inflammation. What emerges is a picture of the body under severe inflammatory stress. Infection or damage has occurred, arthritic or otherwise, and the tissues are doing their best to biochemically communicate their distress. Pain signals and biochemical recruiters are leaping from cell to cell summoning angry white blood cells into the distressed region. Those white blood cells are packing six guns loaded with oxygen free radicals. Those free-radical bullets are fired at perceived threats, and when the bullets hit their targets they busily rip electrons from previously stable molecules to form peculiar, inflexible molecules that behave in eccentric fashion. Sometimes this burst of free-radical oxygen activity is beneficial; liken it to a ray gun of disorder pointed at evil chemical or biological invaders. But sometimes the free-radical balance goes awry, we lose our grip on our own weapon, and the ray gun turns on the good guys.

Eventually, at some point, the old order can no longer exist in the chaos. The old tissue and genetic structure are simply overwhelmed by the intensity and frequency of change. It's like a pot of water that remains steady in its old way as it is gradually heated, but there comes a time when the heat has increased so dramatically that the old order can no longer exist, and a new order—of boiling, dynamic turbulence takes over. There is still an order of sorts, it is just very different; so, too, with a body that gets overheated with inflammation. At some point, for some people, the old order can no longer endure. Change on every level is too dramatic, too dynamic, and a new order arises. Genetic material begins to change, new cells begin to proliferate, and out of the chaos there can emerge a new order. It is called cancer.

When that diseased new order begins to manifest, as cancer competes with the old healthy cellular paradigm, we must consider the wisdom of an old adage: It is possible to blow out a candle, but you can't blow out a fire. If there is some way to blow out the tiny, fragile flame of cancer before it rages, if by reintroducing orderliness within the troubled physiology we could overcome the incipient eruption of chaos, then that is the approach we *must* take. Once the chaos triumphs—once the cancer paradigm gets a strong foothold—then, more dramatic traditional or conventional protocols must be used. But before that biological "sea change" has occurred, the preventative power of herbs and other weapons within the traditional arsenal are the approaches of choice.

CHAPTER FIVE

A Refocus On The Safety of Celebrex and Vioxx

The preceding chapters reveal why both medical professionals and the general public are excited about Celebrex, Vioxx and other potentially selective COX-2 pharmaceuticals. Let's briefly review some of the most recent developments before we look deeper into the issues of safety.

In August 1999, the FDA announced that it would conduct an accelerated "fast track" review of Celebrex to determine if it could *prevent* a rare type of colon cancer. At the same time as the dramatic FDA announcement was made, Monsanto, the developer of Celebrex, announced their collaboration with the National Cancer Institute in initiating human tests of Celebrex for a form of colon cancer, and their plans for other tests to assess the drug's impact on cancers of the skin, esophagus and bladder.

As we noted in the Introduction, as of this writing both Monsanto (the developer of Celebrex) and Merck (the developer of Vioxx) are engaged in extensive clinical testing of the efficacy of Celebrex and Vioxx in preventing colon cancer.

In October 1999, researchers from the M. D. Anderson Cancer Center in Houston, Texas, the National Cancer Institute, and St. Mark's Hospital in England reported that a six-month regimen of Celebrex reduced both the number and size of colorectal polyps in patients with familial adenomatous polyposis. This condition is widely recognized as a precursor to colon cancer. On December 23, 1999, the FDA approved the use of Celebrex as a preventative for those colon polyps.

The excitement over the preventative applications for COX-2 inhibitors continues to grow. For example, on December 30, 1999, researchers from Osaka University reported that by inhibiting COX-2 in tumors that over-expressed that enzyme, those tumors showed reduced growth. Moreover, COX-2 inhibition also reduced the flow of nourishment (through new arterial blood supply) into tumor areas, which also reduced tumor activity and growth. Remember the cancer model: cancers can spread through angiogenesis, or the growth of new blood supply into a region. COX-2 inhibition is thus proven to work on several levels to thwart cancer growth.

In the midst of all this appropriate excitement, we

asked the fundamental question: Are Celebrex and Vioxx safe? This is really a question in two parts: are they safe for *all* people, and are they ideal for *anyone* on a long-term basis? As to the first part, not even the drug manufacturers recommend them for all people, and there are *many* conditions that are contraindications for their use. Of course, that is true for virtually all prescription drugs, and we live with the sobering reality, as reported this year in the *Journal of the American Medical Association*, that over 100,000 people a year die from the unanticipated adverse reactions from taking prescription pharmaceuticals. Nor can we depend on the FDA to thoroughly protect the people of the U.S. from the health threats posed by prescription drugs. As the General Accounting Office of the U.S. Government reported in 1990, more than half of the drugs approved by the FDA have "serious post approval risks including heart failure, birth defects, kidney failure, blindness and convulsions."

A focus on the second part of the question, "Are these drugs a reasonable strategy for anyone on a long-term basis?" also raises serious issues. Medical science was not even aware of the COX-2 enzyme until the early 1990s. Its role and functions in the body, therefore, have not been the subject of extensive long-term consideration. Also, scientists initially thought that the COX-2 enzyme only arose at points and times of inflammation. It was thought to be an artifact or cause of inflammation, an enzyme "induced" by some trauma, insult or injury to the body. In this respect, the "inducible" COX-2 enzyme was thought to be profoundly different from COX-1, which science now believes to be a basic constituent found in nearly all tissues and cells of the body (hence its classification as a "constitutively expressed enzyme").

The preliminary theory that COX-2 was simply an inducible response to inflammation was quickly disproved. Science is coming to understand that COX-2 is also "constitutively" expressed; that is to say, naturally present and presumably performing an ongoing biological function in several organ systems, including the brain and the kidneys. For example, scientists now speculate that COX-2 expression may have a critical role in immune function, in salt, water and body temperature regulation, and in nerve transmission. Besides being induced in cells at points of inflammation, COX-2 is also induced in the ovary and uterus during ovulation and implantation. In a somewhat alarming study on mice, those that had COX-2 totally disabled had an elevated rate of stillbirths due to improper kidney development.

None of this is intended to suggest that persons taking a pharmaceutical COX-2 inhibitor will develop difficulties with brain, reproductive or kidney function. However, it is important to repeat that synthetic COX-2 inhibitors are new, and we do not understand the full range of their activities. Science has only recognized the distinction between COX-1 and COX-2 for less than a decade. We simply don't have enough experience with any pharmaceutical COX-2 inhibitor to be certain, absolutely certain, that it has no dreadful, unintended consequences. The FDA has itself called for additional studies to prove that Celebrex is safer than previously existing NSAIDS. We feel that the answer given by Joan M. Bathon, M.D., of the Johns Hopkins Arthritis Center, captures best the uncertainty surrounding the long-term consequences of a synthetic pharmaceutical COX-2 inhibitor. As reported on the Center's website, Dr. Bathon was posed the simple question: "If COX-2 serves some physiological roles in kidney, brain, and elsewhere, is it wise to selectively inhibit it?" She responded directly: "Until we know the exact function of COX-2 in these organs, this question is not answerable."

Indeed, some of the initial medical establishment euphoria over synthetic COX-2 drugs is wearing off, as Dr. Sandor Szabo of the University of California at Irvine reported at a 1999 meeting of the International Union of Pharmacology. Dr. Szabo was quoted by *Reuter's Health* as stating that the synthetic COX-2 inhibitor drugs "definitely aren't as clean as they were promised to be." Further, he noted that the new class of synthetic COX-2 inhibitors interfered with the healing of gastric ulcers, exacerbated colitis, and might not alleviate the problem of NSAID-related dyspepsia (severe gastric indigestion), which affects 10 to 15% of patients. In other words, while Celebrex, Vioxx and other synthetic COX-2 inhibiting drugs represent a major breakthrough, the jury is still out on the side effects associated with their long-term use.

We feel the need to again affirm our respect for the scientific accomplishments of those who discovered the differential expressions of the COX enzyme systems, and our intellectual respect for the creators of the synthetic chemicals that selectively inhibit COX-2. But, we must reiterate that synthetic, chemical silver bullets that did not previously exist in nature and that target just one molecule in a complex biological process can have serious unanticipated consequences. The very phrasing of that concern impels us to ask: Is there a better, more balanced, more time tested, natural approach to COX-2 inhibition?

CHAPTER SIX

The Confluence of Science and Traditional Medicine

"...how God made the world, a shining plane encircled by the sea,
and through His power established the sun and moon
to light its inhabitants; how he decked the face of the earth
with leaves and branches, and besides gave life to all that moves."
—*Beowulf,* 8th Century C.E.

The world of medical science has appropriately recognized that the discovery of COX-2 is one of the most significant discoveries of the modern era. The dazzling brilliance of this medical discovery should not blind us to the almost ridiculously obvious fact that humankind has just discovered COX-2, this enzyme has functioned from within the DNA of humans and animals since time immemorial. And, if COX-2 has been functioning for aeons, what natural compounds have served to modulate or regulate its dynamic functioning? You see, humans did not inhibit COX-2 one hundred thousand or even five hundred years ago by using a synthetic molecule that targeted unknown manifestations of the enzyme. Human beings tempered and modulated this powerful enzyme with the same complex biochemical, phytochemical tools it used for myriad other biochemical processes. Women and men used herbs.

Do not think for one moment that this herbal intervention was simpleminded or unintended. Traditional medicine has long recognized that people suffer inflammation, and much of traditional medicine is focused on relief from pain and inflammation. In every culture, highly specific herbs, extracted in precise and measured ways, have been employed to modulate inflammation. These ancient phytochemicals are so complex that modern science is only now beginning to understand how they work, and how to make less-than-perfect synthetic copies of them. But then, modern science is only now beginning to speculate on how COX-2 works. One thing is certain, as we will see in the following chapters: the biochemistry of traditional herbs is infinitely more complex, balanced, effective and safe than the silver bullet approach of using one synthetic molecule. Once again, we are not suggesting that the use of the silver bullet is wrong or unnecessary. Indeed, we are confident that it will powerfully and dramatically relieve pain, and likely save many lives. It will almost just as certainly cause pain and suffering and trigger reactions that will cost lives. It is at best one tool, a laser-like molecular weapon that must be considered with care. It is imperative, however, that the far more complex and broadly effective natural COX-2 inhibitors be considered as the first line or complementary treatment for the diseases born of inflammation.

A few notes on the methodology for selecting the COX-2 inhibiting herbs considered in this book. First, we have drawn upon the traditional use of herbs for inflammatory conditions. Second, we have culled from that broad list of traditional herbs the herbs that are either endangered or are not readily available in a high quality form. Third, the herbs that survived the first "cut" were then analyzed by us from two different perspectives. We considered the observed pharmacological effect of the whole herb, and we also considered the pharmacological effects of the principal "phytochemical" constituents of each herb. In other words, we worked both from the whole down to the part, and from the part back to the whole.

In addition to the hundreds of herbal treatises in our own extensive herbal and botanical library, we relied on multiple databases, including most notably the USDA Phytochemical Database, and the University of Illinois Napralert Database. The USDA Database was created and maintained by Dr. James Duke, who is respected as one of the preeminent botanists of our time. The Napralert Database is maintained by Dr. Norman Farnsworth and the Department of Pharmacognosy of the University of Illinois. Dr. Farnsworth is considered one of the fathers of Pharmacognosy, which is the study of plant compounds and their relationship to health and disease. We pay tribute to both of those luminaries, whose research and databases substantially enriched our consideration of COX-2 inhibiting herbs.

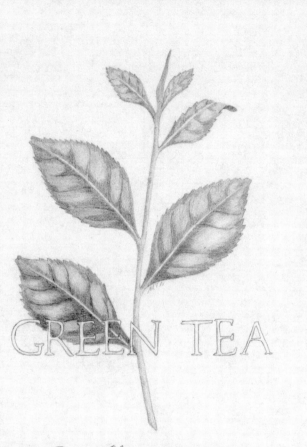

GREEN TEA

Camellia sinensis

CHAPTER SEVEN

Green Tea

THEACEAE, CAMELLIA SINENSIS

Green tea has several highly active COX-2 inhibitors that are worthy of specific mention. It contains salicylic acid, a naturally-occurring COX-2 inhibiting compound that served as the inspiration for acetylsalicylic acid, commonly known as aspirin. Salicylic acid, created from salicin, was first found in nature in the stem bark of the "headache" tree, or the white willow. German scientists almost one hundred years ago added acetic acid to salicylic acid and discovered that it chemically buffered the highly irritating effects of the isolated compound. Thus the beginning of the "Aspirin Century."

As a brief historical digression, the ancient Indian medical system known as Ayurveda ("knowledge of life") employed green tea for many medical conditions, including fever, consistent with green tea's known COX-2 inhibitory effects. The Greek physician Hippocrates discovered, in approximately 400 B.C.E., that chewing on willow bark offered natural pain and fever relief. He probably wrote the Western world's first prescription for a COX-2 inhibitor! Native Americans made a tea from the willow bark as a remedy for headache and rheumatism. Moving forward into more recent times, in 1971 Dr. John Vane demonstrated that acetylsalicylic acid was an inflammatory prostaglandin inhibitor, for which discovery he received the Nobel Prize. Back to green tea . . . .

A recent 1999 study, published in the U.S. Government's *Proceedings of the National Academy of Science*, identifies some of green tea's prominent constituents called polyphenols (GTP) as causing a "marked reduction" in COX-2 induced arthritis. The scientists from Case Western University concluded in this study that a "polyphenolic fraction from green tea that is rich in antioxidants may be useful in the prevention of onset and severity of arthritis." In other research, Swedish scientists located one of these polyphenols, a catechin called flavan-3-ol derivatives, as COX-2 inhibitors. Scientists at the College of Medicine of the National University of Taiwan reported in 1999 that apigenin, another constituent of green tea, was also a "markedly active inhibitor" of COX-2. Parenthetically, German chamomile, *Chamomilla recutita*, also contains apigenin, as well as other biologically active constituents that have preserved this herb's respected place in the herbal pharmacopeia since at least the first century.

Green tea offers two other highly significant features: First, in addition to containing specific COX-2 anti-inflammatories, the Napralert Database reports that green tea contains fifty-one anti-inflammatory compounds. In other words, green tea works as an anti-inflammatory from multiple directions. Second, long-term consumption of tea has been shown to inhibit ulcers that might otherwise be triggered by NSAID use. The *USDA Phytochemical Database* reports that green tea has fifteen anti-ulcer phytonutrients, which is second only to ginger (with seventeen) on its list. Thus, green tea contains compounds that are rich in anti-inflammatory factors that cause a "marked reduction" of COX-2, that prevent the onset and severity of arthritis, *and* that inhibit or prevent ulcers. In contrast, the world is rejoicing that Celebrex and Vioxx offer arthritis pain relief (*not* ulcer prevention), while simply minimizing (maybe) the likelihood of *creating* ulcers. The contrast between the natural and synthetic compounds speaks for itself.

It is important at this point to reflect on the causes of arthritis identified in Chapter Two. You may recall that osteoarthritis is not caused merely by the breakdown of cartilage tissue. It occurs when the cartilage tissue breaks down more quickly (in part due to COX-2 inflammation) than the body is able to heal the wound and replace the cartilage. As we explained, arthritis is a function of the imbalance of the process of destruction and repair. Synthetic COX-2 inhibitors address only the issue of the inflammatory process leading to cartilage deterioration; they were not designed to enhance the body's wound healing or cartilage-repair capabilities. In contrast, the fifteen anti-ulcer phytonutrients in green tea are, by definition, compounds that either prevent wounds or facilitate their healing. This is one of the most important features of natural COX-2 inhibitors—they not only inhibit the inflammatory processes, but natural plant co-factors work to correct the arthritis imbalance by promoting wound healing.

In addition to the anti-arthritic properties of green tea, the most researched health benefit associated with green tea is undoubtedly its anti-cancer effect. Cultures that regularly consume a water extract of green tea have reported a much lower incidence of prostate and other cancers than occur in other developed nations. In a recent study from the Mayo Clinic on green tea consumption and reduction of prostate cancer, it was noted that green tea not only inhibited cancer cell growth, but cancer cells exposed to green tea began to show nuclei fragmentation and other signs of apoptosis, or programmed cell death. What an extraordinary side effect of taking green tea for COX-2 inhibition!

These Mayo Clinic researchers singled out one green tea polyphenol, EGCG, as the most potent inhibitor of cancer cell growth, but they emphasized that green tea's composition is very complex, and they could not identify which specific compound caused the reduction in prostate cancer. Because all of the numerous green tea polyphenols and other compounds are naturally working in concert, it is appropriate to use a broad spectrum extract presenting as complete a representation of the plant's constituents as possible.

This is a good occasion to emphasize again the value of a broad-spectrum extract. While the Mayo clinic researchers identified one particular green tea polyphenol, EGCG, as having the greatest anti-tumor activity, Japanese medical researchers reported in 1998 that the "non-phenolic fraction has potent suppressive activities against tumor promotion." This is not to say that the catechin EGCG doesn't have potent anti-tumor properties, it is just that the wisdom of the whole herb cannot be ignored. Similarly, two recent studies from Rutgers University concluded that the caffeine in green tea somehow played an important role in activating the herb's anti-tumor properties. It is not the polyphenols alone. It is not the *non*-polyphenols alone. It is not the green tea caffeine alone. It is all of the myriad compounds naturally present in the herb, taken and acting in concert, that have caused green tea to be revered by both traditional medicine and newly appreciated by modern science. Frankly, green tea is a powerhouse of known and yet to be discovered COX-2 inhibitors.

With regard to how to best consume a beneficial amount of green tea, the traditional way is to sip green tea throughout the day. It is believed that drinking four or more standard cups of green tea will provide a beneficial dosage of the plant's phytonutrients. For many of you, drinking four or more cups of green tea may not comfortably fit within the tradition of your daily routine. In such circumstances, you should consider supplementing with an appropriate green tea extract. Later in the book we will offer guidelines for selecting appropriate extracts. But, at this juncture, it is enough to suggest that an extract of green tea should mimic, as closely as possible, the constituents in the traditional form of green tea consumption. As green tea was traditionally consumed using a water extract—a simple cup of tea— we recommend using a water extract for this herb.

Finally, just as the compounds *within* green tea are complex and synergistic, green tea polyphenols show a marked synergy with other herbs, particularly with respect to anti-tumor activity. For example, combining the polyphenol EGCG from green tea with the curcuminoids from turmeric (or logically from ginger, a related species and similar source of curcumin) resulted in a threefold increase in the anti-tumor properties of curcumin, and an eightfold increase in the anti-tumor properties of EGCG. Accordingly, we recommend that green tea extracts be broad-spectrum and be used in combination with extracts of turmeric and ginger.

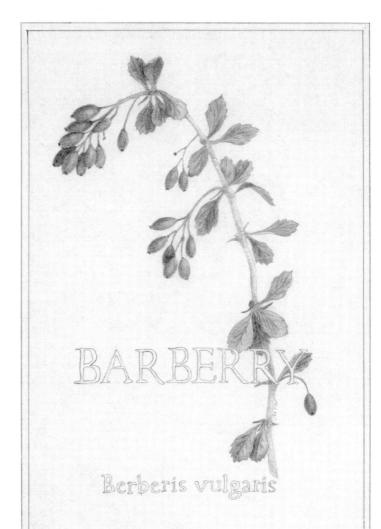

BARBERRY

Berberis vulgaris

CHAPTER EIGHT

Chinese Goldthread and Barberry

RANUNCULACEAE, COPTIS CHINENSIS (HUANG LIAN)
BERBERIDACEAE, BERBERIS VULGARIS

Both Chinese goldthread (native to the mountains of China, particularly the Szechwan province) and barberry (native to Europe and naturalized in North America) are rich natural sources of a substance called berberine. Berberine is bright yellow in appearance, and is somewhat bitter. It has been used in traditional medicine for its anti-inflammatory and anti-microbial effects. In ancient Egypt, berries from barberry were mixed with fennel to treat fevers, and the Catawba Indians, of the region of North America now the Carolinas, used barberry for peptic ulcers. In Bulgaria and throughout Eastern Europe, root extracts of the *Berberidaceae* species were used in rheumatic and other chronic inflammatory disorders. These traditional herbal uses for inflammation and fever confirm historically what science has now established in the laboratory: Compounds in these plants inhibit the COX-2 enzyme.

A 1999 article published in the *Journal of Ethnopharmacology* confirmed that berberine found in barberry and Chinese goldthread inhibits COX-2. The study further confirms that COX-2 is "abundantly expressed in colon cancer cells and plays a role in tumorigenesis . . . ." The berberine/COX-2 connection "may further explain the mechanism of anti-inflammatory and anti-tumor promoting effects of berberine." In 1998 research from Japan, Chinese goldthread and its constituent berberine were found to suppress colon carcinogenesis and to inhibit COX-2 without also inhibiting COX-1. In other words, berberine is a selective COX-2 inhibitor. Research from the College of Medicine of the National University of Taiwan published in 1999 further identified kaempferol, another constituent of barberry, as a "markedly active inhibitor" of COX-2. A recent report from the China Medical College of Taiwan explained that berberine supported the eradication of human bladder tumors. Another wonderful side effect of taking an herbal COX-2 inhibitor!

But that is not the end of the berberine story. Consider the following three studies:

• Yang Ming Medical College of Taiwan reported in 1995 that berberine induced the apoptosis or cellular suicide of human leukemia cells;

• The journal *Oncology* reported in 1986 that berberine inhibited skin tumor formation;

• The Hebei Medical College of Shiziazhaung, China, reported in 1990 that berberine has "potent anti-tumor activity against human and rat malignant brain tumors."

Berberine-containing herbs thus offer significant medical benefits across the spectrum of diseases.

As is clear from our discussion of green tea, we believe in the intelligence and healing power of the *whole* herb, and strongly prefer full spectrum extracts to a pharmacological isolation of only one ingredient. The research on the anti-inflammatory properties of barberry again confirms the wisdom of the whole herb approach. Researchers at the Institute of Microbiology from the Bulgarian Academy of Sciences tested the anti-inflammatory capabilities of a full-spectrum extract of barberry versus five of its other active fractions.

Note: All of the isolates and the composite alkaloid fractions are part of the full-spectrum, total herb extract. Each of the extracts was applied in acute inflammation, and the full- spectrum or total herb extract demonstrated the greatest anti-inflammatory effect. The researchers also discovered that the full-spectrum total herb extract was most effective in reducing the inflammation associated with an arthritic condition. It was not that the other fractions did not work to reduce inflammation—they just weren't as effective as the total herb extract. There is a brilliance to berberine, but there is greater genius in using the COX-2 inhibitory effects of berberine in the context of the full plant.

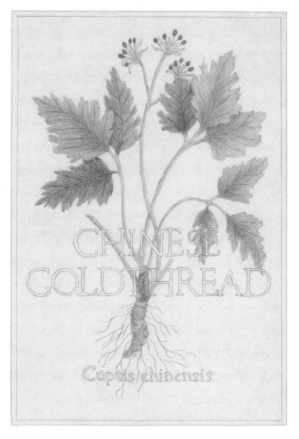

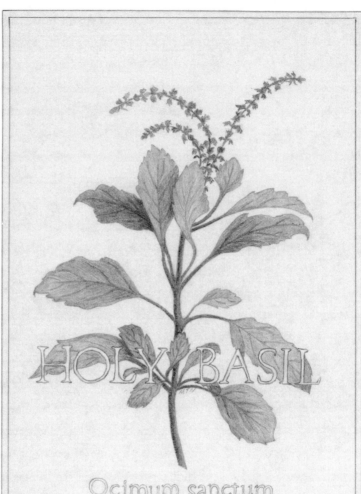

HOLY BASIL

Ocimum sanctum

CHAPTER NINE

Holy Basil

LABIATAE, OCIMUM SANCTUM (TULSI)

Holy basil is so named because of the tradition of planting this herb around the temple courtyards of India. It is said to be the herb sacred to the goddess Lakshmi and her divine husband Vishnu, the Hindu deities responsible for maintaining balance in life and creation. Its Hindi name, *tulsi*, means "matchless," indicative of its exalted status in traditional Ayurvedic medicine. Holy basil is indigenous to India, but is now cultivated throughout Central and South America for its medicinal properties.

Ocimum sanctum, otherwise known as holy basil (not the same as common, culinary basil or *Ocimum basilicum*), contains phytonutrients that have "significant COX-2 inhibitory effect." The phytonutrient "ursolic acid" is specifically recognized for its COX-2 inhibitory effects. In research conducted at the Dartmouth Medical School, a study confirmed that derivatives of oleanolic acid and ursolic acid possessed potential anti-inflammatory and cancer-preventing activity related to their inhibition of COX-2. One recent French study identified ursolic acid as a causative agent in the "programmed" cell death of human leukemia cells. The above studies, together with numerous other recent studies from around the world, reflect *Ocimum sanctum*'s recognized role as both an inhibitor of COX-2 and of an enzymatic cousin of COX-2, lipoxygenase.

As often repeated in this analysis, the great problem with NSAIDS, and an emerging concern with synthetic COX-2 inhibitors, is their ulcerative effect. Just as with green tea, *Ocimum sanctum* has scientifically confirmed anti-ulcerative properties. In a 1993 study from India, even a seven-day treatment of *Ocimum sanctum* had significant anti-ulcer effects. In addition, there is substantial scientific confirmation that *Ocimum sanctum* is antimutagenic, radioprotective, possesses significant anti-tumor effects in human skin and increases a key detoxification enzyme called glutathione S-transferase activity. No wonder that this herb is deemed sacred in India and is in widespread use throughout the world.

A final note: the research on holy basil's radioprotective properties is impressive. The term "radioprotective" describes the herb's ability to protect the DNA of the body from the dangerous, mutating power of various forms of radiation. We are assaulted by the destabilizing influence of radiation in many ways and at many different levels of intensity. The daily effect of exposure to sunlight provides one type of radiation; at the other extreme is the profound assault that accompanies conventional radiation therapy. One of the real problems with radiation damage is that it is cumulative. With every additional moment of excess exposure to the sun, with every trip through a metal detection machine in an airport, and with every exposure to discrete bursts of higher intensity radiation from other sources, our cells absorb and store the cumulative destabilizing inflammatory effects. At a certain point, the DNA becomes so weary from absorbing the repeated blows that, like a tired fighter in the fifteenth round, it just collapses. The collapse of the orderliness and intelligence of DNA is a profoundly grave threat to the health of our cells and our body. To prevent such a genetic disaster, we urge you on an individual level, and oncologists on behalf of the medical establishment, to incorporate this radioprotective herb at tonic levels in daily life and at therapeutic levels in circumstances of radiation therapy.

The use of holy basil will not protect us from exposure to radiation insult, but it will offer a form of protection. To take our boxing analogy one more step, holy basil offers a way to strengthen our natural defense mechanisms, much like wearing protective headgear, which allows us to withstand the radiation "punches" more effectively. And this form of protection is so easy to obtain! Therefore, we believe that this herb must be included in everyone's program of preventative medicine.

We recommend an extract of this herb that is marked for the presence of ursolic acid, the constituent that has confirmed COX-2 inhibitory properties.

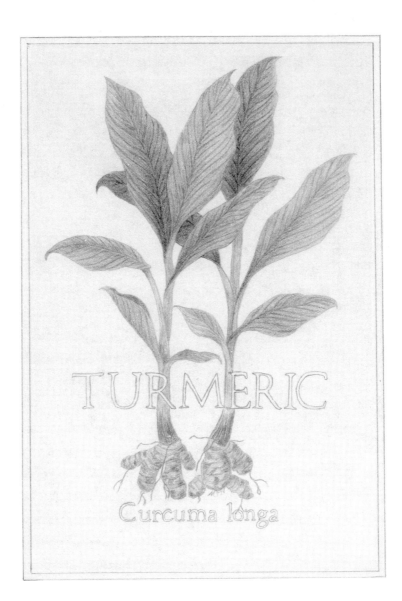

TURMERIC

Curcuma longa

CHAPTER TEN

Turmeric

ZINGIBERACEAE, CURCUMA LONGA
(*HALDI* IN HINDI, *JIANG HUANG* IN CHINESE)

"Curcuma...Turmerick, the root opens the Gall...cures the Jaundies."
1671, Salmon, *Syn. Med.*

An entire book could easily, and justifiably, be written on the scientifically confirmed healing properties of turmeric. This cousin of ginger, part of the *Zingiberaceae* family and indigenous to India and southern Asia, was long thought by the West to be merely a humble coloring agent or food additive. Much more, turmeric rhizome extract demonstrates powerful anti-inflammatory properties, is extraordinarily anti-oxidative, inhibits the life-threatening process by which fat in the body becomes rancid, and consistently exhibits pronounced anti-tumor properties. It is widely used in traditional Ayruvedic and Chinese medical systems for, among other purposes, the stimulation of beneficial liver action and to relieve digestive inflammation.

Researchers from New York Presbyterian Hospital and the Weill Medical College of Cornell University reported in their 1999 article in *Cancer Research* that curcumin, a major phytochemical in the bright orange root of the turmeric plant, directly inhibited the activity of COX-2. The authors concluded that "these data provide new insights into the anti-cancer properties of curcumin." For example, researchers at Vanderbilt University in 1999 reported that turmeric inhibits TxA2, which in turn indicates that COX-2 has been inhibited. As discussed above, TxA2 participates in or facilitates angiogenesis, which is the growth of new blood vessels into regions of tumor proliferation. In other words, phytonutrients in turmeric inhibit the mechanism that creates the blood supply needed for tumor growth. Turmeric has been identified as a colon cancer suppressor and an inhibitor of skin cancer. As the journal *Cancer Research* concluded, this demonstrated cancer inhibiting capability is attributed "at least in part, to the modulation of arachidonic acid [Omega-6] metabolism." That, as explained above, is where both COX-1 and COX-2 work to create inflammatory hormones in the body.

The precise way in which curcumin and turmeric inhibit COX-2 is the subject of continuing serious study, but one recent report, in the October 1999 issue of the journal *Oncogene,* gives a sense of the remarkable discrimination and precise effect of the curcumin constituent. No one will be quizzed on the following; it is described only to reveal that the biochemical activity is precise, measurable and complex. The researchers from the University of Leicester, England, explained that in human colon cells, curcumin inhibited COX-2 induction by preventing the "phosphorylation of IkappaB by inhibiting the activity of the IKKs."

Just to give you a glimpse of some of the recognized benefits of curcumin, as reflected in hundreds of published scientific papers:

- More DNA protective than lipoate, vitamin E and beta carotene
- Stimulates glutathione S-transferase, a detoxifying, cancer-protective enzyme
- Modulates nitric oxide and is associated with its anti-inflammatory and anti-cancer activities
- Strongly anti-inflammatory, both orally and topically, and, like green tea and *Ocimum sanctum*, is anti-ulcerative
- Intensifies the anti-cancer activity of other phytonutrients
- Inhibits leukemia at initiation, promotion and progression
- Inhibits precancerous colon lesions

71

- Inhibits the growth of multiple breast cancer cell lines
- Suppresses colon cancer
- Inhibitory of oral tumors
- Topically applied curcumin can strongly inhibit skin tumor promotion.

We thus do not minimize the importance of curcumin, but we caution against using turmeric extracts that are standardized to such a high concentration of curcumin that the extract takes on a pharmaceutical nature. Those silver-bullet curcumin extracts miss the complex value of the total herb, and we believe that scientific research is clearly demonstrating that the full spectrum of this powerful herb, with all its phytochemical notes, tones and nuances, is the best way to derive maximum benefit. Consider this when you are tempted by a straight curcumin extract: In 1997, a scientific study demonstrated that a curcumin-free extract possessed more powerful anti-tumor activity than the dried herb or a straight alcohol extract, both of which contained some aspects of curcumin. Similarly, a 1998 study reported that a curcumin-free water extract offered significant protection against breast cancer. Several recent studies also report that water extracts of turmeric contain antimutagenic activities comparable to pure curcumin. Accordingly, we would be concerned that a highly isolated turmeric extract standardized only to curcumin would miss the recognized cancer-preventive and anti-inflammatory properties present in the whole plant. We would also be concerned if the extract method selected failed to extract curcumin together with the full spectrum of other turmeric constituents. Again, nature has selected the compounds bundled in turmeric, and we don't counsel substituting our limited judgment for that of millions of years of natural processes, and thousands of years of safe and effective use of turmeric's broad spectrum of ingredients.

LOOKING FOR A TONIC LEVEL THAT IS "JUST RIGHT"

We sound one other important note of caution regarding a pure curcumin extract. We have expressed our concern about the unknown effects of the silver bullet of *synthetic* COX-2 chemicals. Similarly, we are concerned about the unknown effects of the silver-bullet approach of the *natural* COX-2 inhibitors. Pumping just one isolated molecule into our bodies, even one extracted from a revered herb, exposes the physiology to both unknown risk and incomplete benefit. In nature, the potency of one phytonutrient is always buffered and balanced by other protective compounds in the herb. The caffeine in green tea, for example, is clearly a stimulant, but it is buffered by other soothing phytonutrients in the

73

herb that take the edge off the caffeine's stimulating effects. Ironically, removing the caffeine from green tea appears to deactivate green tea's powerful anti-tumor effects. Now consider curcumin alone, in a concentrated form, without turmeric's natural buffers. The turmeric plant, in its natural state, is an anti-oxidant. That means that all of the constituents of turmeric, working together, reduce the potentially tumor-causing and aging effects of free oxygen radicals in the body. If curcumin is isolated out of the plant—which means the isolate is no longer turmeric, but is now a pharmaceutical chemical— curcumin can actually increase the damaging effects of free radicals of oxygen. Scientists use a word to describe a compound that is beneficial at one level but dangerous at another. That term is "biphasic," and curcumin is a classic expression of a biphasic compound. At low levels, such as naturally exists in the context of the whole turmeric rhizome, curcumin is extraordinarily beneficial. In a highly concentrated and unnaturally isolated form, curcumin can be problematic. For example, where full spectrum turmeric stimulates a cancer detoxification enzyme called glutathione S-transferase (GST), high doses of isolated curcumin may suppress GST. One isolated chemical constituent of an herb, like curcumin, can thus have exactly the opposite effect of the full spectrum herb.

In this way, a pure curcumin extract acts like an over-dose of synthetic vitamin C, known as ascorbic acid. In intelligent amounts, vitamin C is an important anti-oxidant, which people should derive from their foods and from whole food supplements. But taking large doses of ascorbic acid, a synthetic chemical isolate, can actually stimulate the potential for free-radical damage. Yes, ascorbic acid is simply a synthetic form of vitamin C, but you can't assume that a synthetic vitamin isolate taken in large, pharmacological doses is always beneficial.

Consider the similar issue with calcium mega-supplementation. Women are being exhorted to take huge dosages of supplemental calcium, on the theory that dumping calcium carbonate into the physiology will somehow strengthen a woman's bones during and after menopause. Adding calcium carbonate to the diet, which is the exact chemical equivalent of eating chalk, is a curious idea to begin with, but what are the possible downsides to such mega-supplementation? First, in many cases of arthritis you will find tiny chemical crystals in the joints. These crystals may be irritants or sources of pain, and they are comprised of . . . that's right, calcium. So, the very thing people are taking to minimize osteoporosis may be actually exacerbating arthritis. And are megadoses of chemical calcium absorbed and used by the body? Research published in the *Annals of Internal Medicine* showed a stark contrast between calcium taken as part of the normal diet and megadose calcium in the form of chalk. The more calcium the women took in the form of chalk, the higher the incidence of kidney stones; the more calcium in the form of food, the lower the incidence of kidney stones. Such is the wisdom of whole food.

Forgive the analogy, but the story of Goldilocks comes to mind. The body, like Goldilocks, does not thrive on things too hot, too cold, too hard or too soft, but instead benefits from "just right." The therapeutic dosage of "just rightness" is the goal, and more often than not that proper balance comes from using the natural tools of food and herbs.

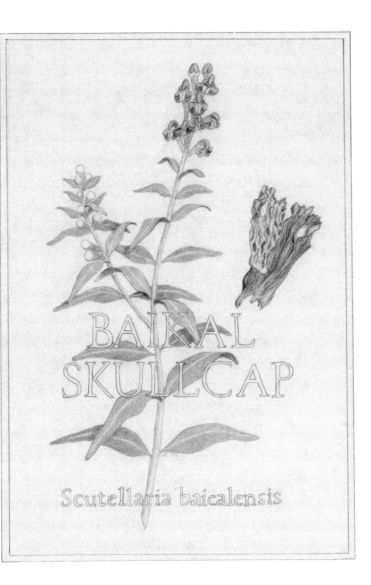

BAIKAL
SKULLCAP

Scutellaria baicalensis

CHAPTER ELEVEN

Baikal Skullcap

LAABIATAE, SCUTELLARIA BAICALENSIS

This herb is commonly known in the West as both *Scutellaria baicalensis* and Baikal skullcap, and in Chinese herbalism, as *Huang Qin*. *Scutellaria* is native to China, Japan, Korea, Mongolia and parts of Russia. The root of this herb, harvested from three- to four-year-old plants, is a rich source of a well-researched flavonoid called baicalein. This herb is long revered in Chinese medicine, as confirmed from its inclusion in ancient writings (on wooden tablets) found in a second century tomb in north-western China. The herb was traditionally used for high fevers, consistent with our current understanding that baicalein inhibits COX-2.

In research from Barcelona University in Spain published in 1999, scientists determined that baicalein inhibits COX-2. Recent experimental results from Japan also demonstrated that *Scutellaria* suppressed colon cancer, which is consistent with *Scutellaria's* inhibition of COX-2. Scientists around the world are accelerating laboratory research on this impressive botanical. For example, Korean scientists discovered in 1998 that *Scutellaria* stimulated the creation of an important cancer detoxification enzyme called quinone reductase. Two compounds from *Scutellaria* substantially inhibit skin tumors. Previous scientific research out of Korea reported that *Scutellaria* demonstrated both anti-inflammatory and wound healing properties, and research in the Ukraine demonstrated that this herb inhibited lipoxygenase metabolism of arachidonic acid, the benefits of which were touched upon briefly in the chapter on green tea and will be explored in more detail in the ginger discussion. It is important to once again observe that *Scutellaria* has demonstrated both COX-2 anti-inflammatory properties and powerful wound healing effects. In what is something of a *mantra* in this book, we repeat that the diseases of arthritis and other inflammatory conditions are diseases of imbalance. The majesty of an herb like *Scutellaria* lies in its ability to restore physiological balance both by inhibiting COX-2 inflammation and promoting the healing of damaged tissue through its wound-healing properties.

Now, for a little medical speculation. As we

explained in Chapter Four, nitric oxide is produced at the point of inflammation, and is now thought to be a factor in the formation and growth of cancers. As we readily acknowledged in that same chapter, no one knows precisely what nitric oxide does, but the association between peaks of nitric oxide production and cancer is becoming clear. It turns out that baicalein, and a sister compound in *Scutellaria* called "wogonin," inhibited the creation of nitric oxide. Wogonin actually appears to be even a stronger inhibitor of nitric oxide than baicalein, which is yet another piece of evidence in support of using the whole herb. The point of this is that *Scutellaria* works to reduce and control inflammation in many ways, some understood and some beyond the current grasp of Western science. It is fascinating, however, that humble *Scutellaria* contained multiple nitric oxide inhibitors for perhaps millions of years before we even discovered nitric oxide in the body. We should, in fairness to turmeric, ginger and *hu zhang*, also note that the phytochemicals curcumin (contained in both ginger and turmeric) and resveratrol (contained in *hu zhang*, as you will read in the next chapter) also scavenge or inhibit nitric oxide. Interesting how the pieces start to fall together: COX-2 and nitric oxide are discovered within only the past few years, and the traditional herbs have been here all along, waiting to be discovered again and put to work.

The consideration of *Scutellaria* in this book is, on one hand, obvious: it contains at least one compound known to inhibit COX-2, and a related compound has been shown to suppress colon cancer. On the other hand, we have already recommended multiple compounds in green tea, turmeric and holy basil as COX-2 inhibitors, as we will continue to do with other herbs. Why the multiplicity of COX-2 inhibitors? That's simple. The little that is known of COX-2 tells us that the enzyme's activity is astonishingly complex. We now understand that COX-1 and COX-2 are both necessary in some levels and proportions to support health. To strike a knock-out blow to COX-2 via one synthetic compound seems to ignore the real issue or problem with COX-2 imbalance, and that is where the wisdom of nature comes into play. Traditional medicine views the herbs considered here as "modulators," restoring balance more than striking a lethal blow. With most of the herbal COX-2 inhibitors we are recommending, we find that the herbs inhibit COX-2 *while at the same time providing significant digestive protection and wound healing effects.* Not only do many of these herbs reduce inflammation, they support stomach and intestinal functions, are anti-ulcerative and strongly promote wound healing.

Conversely, there are toxicities associated with synthetic compounds, while there are buffers, synergies and protective aspects when dealing with a complex of herbs. One herb, like turmeric, supports and magnifies the efficacy of green tea, while another COX-2 inhibitor approaches that enzyme from a slightly different direction. There is, after all, not just one COX-2 herbal inhibitor in nature's apothecary, so we believe that using the herbs in concert is taking fullest advantage of nature's wisdom. In traditional medicine, it is customary to allow herbs to work together. In a way, it is a fail-safe mechanism. If *Scutellaria* is not the COX-2 inhibitor that works for a particular person, then the inhibitory properties of turmeric or green tea can step in and fulfill this critical function.

Does this mean that these COX-2 inhibiting herbs are not as immediate or overwhelming in their effect as their synthetic pharmaceutical counterparts? There is one possible explanation, and one that would be advanced by proponents of the synthetic approach. But, it is more likely that the herbs work in a natural way, harmonious with our physiology, safely and gently balancing and supporting the body as it works to reduce inflammation, promote wound healing and thereby restore balance in our lives.

There is one other important point that people want to forget when confronted with discomfort or pain. Inflammation, that cell-to-cell signal of pain, is a way of directing the mind and body to the point of distress. It is nature's way of requiring us to address and remedy a problem. If there's a rock in our shoe, the pain tells us in no uncertain terms that we need to remove it. If our joint cartilage is damaged, the pain tells us that we cannot put stress on that joint without causing more damage. So, when we have pain, inflammatory compounds direct, in still mysterious ways, the flow of intelligence in the body to the point of pain. Blood, with all its healing and cleansing properties, is rushing to the inflamed site. The mind is drawn, indeed compelled, to think about the pain. That is the way of nature, as if to insist that the mind and body cooperate to resolve the problem. When our full mental and physical resources are summoned and working together, broken bones *do* heal, ulcers *can* go away, damaged skin and flesh *can* regenerate, and cancerous cells *are destroyed* every day.

On the other hand, we are not masochists, and there comes a time when the pain overshadows and we are so gripped by it that we cannot function. That is why people have taken NSAIDS for decades. While there does come a time to blunt pain's sharp knife, to simply blast an area into oblivion, to anesthetize a pocket or joint of pain, offers a limited scope of pain relief. The better approach, to us, is to use the wisdom of herbs to achieve intelligent, balanced reduction of inflammation, and then take other steps to promote the deeper healing that needs to occur. Some of the herbs discussed here actually work on these deeper levels, and stimulate or activate that healing. By contrast, synthetic COX-2 inhibitors and other NSAIDS make no claim to promote the deeper healing. At best, the new super-aspirins *hope* to minimize harm, and the jury is nervously undecided on their success.

Scutellaria offers yet another potent reason to use an herbal "complex" rather than a "silver bullet." The root of this plant (the part we have recommended) has been used in China for thousands of years to treat inflammation and allergies. A Chinese scientist at the University of Chicago had an interest in studying this herb, and he and a number of his colleagues discovered that *Scutellaria's* anti-oxidant molecules had just the right shape to quickly slip inside cellular membranes. In a demonstration of the cleverness, if not genius, of these researchers, someone made the association to a particular problem related to cardiac arrest. In a heart attack, the cells are deprived of oxygen and energy, and toxins build up rapidly within the heart tissue. When the blockage shifts and some oxygen is restored, the cells begin a rapid emergency cleaning campaign, analogous to the clean-ups that occur in the aftermath of a hurricane. During this frenzy of toxin removal, there is a severe and rapid build-up of reactive oxygen, or free radicals. Ironically, the very action needed to clean up the toxic damage results in a different kind of toxicity, and often the cells cannot survive with such a concentration of free radicals. The result: heart tissue dies, and death can quickly occur. Such a death by free-radical poisoning is one model of a fatal heart attack.

These same researchers understood that the molecules of free-radical scavengers, such as vitamins C and E, bind to free radicals, thus inactivating them. The problem, referred to above, was that in a heart attack the damage happens so quickly that the vitamin C and E scavengers can't get inside the cell walls quickly enough, and thus can't rescue the tissue from permanent damage. The scientists thought that the molecular shape of *Scutellaria* would allow its molecules to quickly penetrate the cell membranes, and they devised a simple test. They simulated a human heart attack in the similar heart tissue of a chicken, to see if the *Scutellaria* molecules could "slip in." As anticipated, the herb's free radical scavengers quickly gained entry through the cellular membranes and significantly abated the tissue damage. Under these extreme circumstances of a simulated cardiac arrest, it is not surprising that there was still some cellular damage, but the cells regained enough function to support normal muscular activity and life.

If that's not enough, it appears that *Scutellaria* inhibits compounds that are an integral part of the pancreatic cancer process. Researchers from Creighton University School of Medicine reported in 1999 that baicalein induced apoptosis, or the cellular suicide, of four pancreatic cell types. Baicalein, one of the best-researched constituents of *Scutellaria*, destroyed pancreatic cancer cells by taking away their specific high-octane food source.

Finally, researchers from the University of Guelph in Canada reported in the prestigious British Medical Journal, *The Lancet,* that *Scutellaria* also contains high concentrations of melatonin, a hormone produced by the pineal gland that has significant known anti-cancer effects. One of the many beneficial effects of melatonin is that it is another inhibitor of the enzyme pathway that creates fuel for cancer cells. So with *Scutellaria*, with the whole herb, we can reap the benefits of two proven inhibitors of potentially dangerous metabolic pathways.

The moral of this story: With a synthetic silver bullet you get one specific molecular activity. After all, these are designer molecules, and they were manufactured to disrupt or inhibit just one process. But nature is more economical, more efficient with its biochemical resources. With the natural intricacy of a complex botanical, which nature designed to exist in a world of multiple threats and challenges, the herbs have "multitasking" capabilities. You take *Scutellaria* for its anti-inflammatory and anti-cancer COX-2 inhibiting effects, and *Lo!*, you are also receiving the services of a "SWAT team" of free-radical scavengers far more effective than vitamins C or E, and cancer-fuel inhibitors that protect organs like the pancreas from mortal peril. This is the glory of using a natural substance.

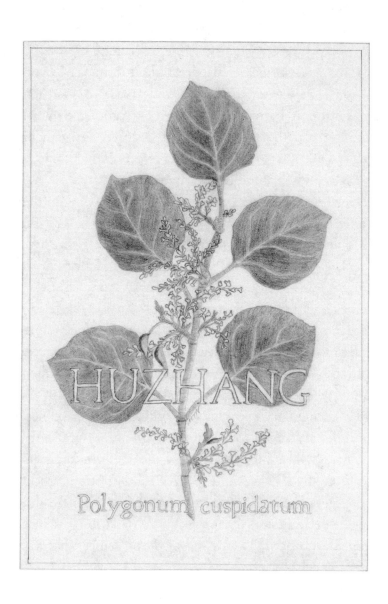

HUZHANG

Polygonum cuspidatum

CHAPTER TWELVE

Hu zhang (Japanese Knotweed)
POLYGONACEAE, POLYGONUM CUSPIDATUM

This herb, native to Japan, has stems up to six and one-half feet tall that resemble bamboo, with rounded leaves and cream flowers. Like ginger and turmeric, *hu zhang* is born of a rhizome, and in Chinese medicine both the leaves and the rhizome are used. A root decoction is typically used to make an anti-arthritic wash, consistent with its COX-2 inhibiting capabilities. *Hu zhang* is a member of the polygonum family, which is known generally in the West as Solomon's Seal. It is not known why this and other herbs in this family are called, in the Western world, Solomon's Seal, but it is interesting to note the ancient words of King Solomon:

[God] himself gave me true understanding of things as they are: a knowledge of the structure of the world and the operation of the elements; the beginning and end of epochs and their middle course; the alternating solstices and changing seasons; the cycles of the years and the constellations; the nature of living creatures and behavior of wild beasts; the violent force of winds and the thoughts of men; the varieties of plants and the virtues of roots.

Perhaps King Solomon was aware of the healing powers of the family of plants later to bear his name, but modern scientists clearly understand that one plant within that family, *hu zhang*, contains a powerhouse constituent called "resveratrol." That discovery was documented by scientists in 1993 at Purdue University. It has since been determined that *hu zhang* is nature's richest known source of resveratrol, even though red grapes, and the wines made thereof, have of late received more attention for containing this compound.

Parenthetically, a lovely consideration of this other and more famous resveratrol-containing plant can be found in Dr. James Duke's recent work, *Herbs of the Bible*, where Dr. Duke observes that resveratrol is "a stress metabolite present in grape leaves and grape skins," and that it is a cyclooxygenase inhibitor. Dr. Duke suggests that a meal of grape leaves, spiced with turmeric and pepper, and stuffed with rice (one of the resveratrol-rich cereals), would have anti-arthritic, anti-cancer, and heart protective qualities. We commend this wonderful book for your further enrichment.

What is the importance of resveratrol? Scientists at Memorial Sloan-Kettering Cancer Center reported in 1998 that resveratrol is a powerful suppressor of COX-2 cancer promotion. The authors of the report concluded that this COX-2 inhibition is "likely to be important for understanding the anti-cancer and anti-inflammatory properties of resveratrol." More recently, scientists at the University of Illinois Department of Surgical Oncology reported that resveratrol inhibits COX-2 and "restores glutathione levels (supporting cancer detoxification in the liver)" as well as stimulates the production of powerful and natural free-radical scavengers. In a major collaboration of researchers from the Memorial Sloan-Kettering Cancer Center, Cornell Medical Center and several other prestigious institutions, scientists determined that resveratrol "directly inhibits the activity of COX-2" in human breast cancer cells and malignant oral tissue. Resveratrol accomplished this by performing two extraordinarily complex and difficult to understand feats: (1) it inhibited the cellular expression of the COX-2 gene; and (2) it inhibited the actual enzyme activity of COX-2. Interesting that something so simple as a red grape or the *hu zhang* root can perform such complex biochemical activities. This is the quiet genius of nature.

Accordingly, we believe that an herbal COX-2 inhibition approach should incorporate this rich source of resveratrol, which has demonstrable antioxidant and anti-tumor properties. (And, after taking the appropriate herbal supplement, some of you may want to savor a glass of red wine as a liquid resveratrol supplement!)

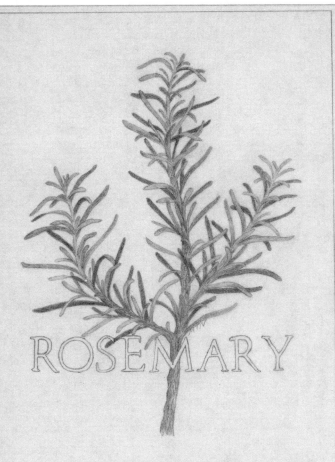

ROSEMARY

Rosmarinus officinalis

CHAPTER THIRTEEN

Rosemary

LAMIACEAE, ROSMARINUS OFFICINALIS

As for Rosemarine, I lett it runne all over my garden walls,
not onlie because my bees love it, but because it is the herb
sacred to remembrance, and, therefore, to friendship . . . .
—Sir Thomas More

Rosemary is native to the Mediterranean, growing
freely throughout much of southern Europe, and is now
cultivated and adored worldwide. Its Latin name,
Rosmarinus, means "sea dew," referring to its natural
habitat. It enjoys the deep respect of European herbal
medicine, where it is regularly used to improve concentration and memory and to relieve headache. Applied
topically, the oils of rosemary continue to be used to
relieve aching, rheumatic muscles.

In 1992, before the fireworks began on COX-2,
researchers at the Faculte de Medecine, Universite de

Limoges, France, reported that ursolic acid, a constituent of both *Ocimum sanctum* and rosemary, inhibited arachidonic acid metabolism in human platelet and leukemia cells. Then, in 1994, researchers at Rutgers University determined that rosemary extracts inhibited a number of processes that are known to fuel the growth of tumors. How significantly did rosemary inhibit these dangerous activities? According to the Rutgers researchers, by up to ninety-nine percent. Confirming our strong preference for the whole herb, the Rutgers scientists determined that two of rosemary's constituents, ursolic acid and carnosol, also demonstrated inhibitory effects on these pernicious processes, but the inhibition was not as dramatic as that demonstrated by the whole plant.

Specific confirmation of the rosemary—COX-2 relationship was unearthed in 1998 by Swedish scientists who identified ursolic acid, a major component of rosemary (and, of course, of *Ocimum sanctum*) as possessing a "significant COX-2 inhibitory effect." Another rosemary constituent, apigenin, was subsequently identified in 1999 by researchers at the National University of Taiwan as a "markedly active inhibitor" of COX-2. Similarly, at Dartmouth Medical School, an ongoing intensive search continues for patentable COX-2 inhibitors, among eighty novel compounds, all of which are derived from oleanolic and ursolic acid, constituents of rosemary.

NOW, FOR A BRIEF
PHILOSOPHICAL DIGRESSION

We appreciate the zeal of the Dartmouth researchers. From their research and from other similar explorations around the world, scientists may yet uncover just the pharmaceutical silver bullet that will, with one shot, disable the COX-2 pathway with no adverse side effects. But we suspect not. The problem with searching for that one patentable silver bullet, whether it is Celebrex, Vioxx, or something new, is that such a silver-bullet approach assumes that the body and mind work in a linear, predictable way. This fictitious linearity was beautifully exposed and debunked by Dr. Arnold Mandell, whose insights were reported in the book *Chaos* by James Gleick. Dr. Mandell critiqued modern psychopharmacology for its consistent failures, and he attributed these failures to a gross oversimplification of the activities of the body and mind. Gleick quotes Dr. Mandell as stating that the "underlying paradigm remains: one gene ➔ one peptide ➔ one enzyme ➔ one neurotransmitter ➔ one receptor ➔ one animal behavior ➔ one clinical syndrome ➔ one drug ➔ one clinical rating scale."

Such a linear model of the body as it expresses itself in the brain was, to Dr. Mandell, profoundly unprofound, almost naïve. "More than 50 transmitters, thousands of cell types, complex electromagnetic phenomenology, and continuous instability based autonomous activity at all levels, from proteins to the electroencephalogram—and still the brain is thought of as a chemical point-to-point switchboard." Mandell did not see a straight line: he saw, according to Gleick, "flowing geometries that sustain complex systems like the mind."

And that is what we are, a flowing geometry. That is the essence of our ever-changing physical reality. You take da Vinci's famous drawing of a man, arms and legs outstretched within a square within a circle. Entitled *Vitruvian Man*, it is a powerful image that has long gripped our imaginations. But now let's make it real: spin that circle in three dimensions, change its locations in time and space, subject it to aging, decaying, radiation, heat, wind, hormones, stress, heartbeats, breaths and myriad foods. Watch as it regenerates, reproduces and dies. You've seen such a picture before: it is the image of our lives. In the midst of that magnificent impermanence, is it even remotely possible that the COX-2 enzyme process is simple and linear? Can anyone really believe for a moment that we can reduce the COX-2 enzyme process to a static "pathway" that is a straight line, and that we can simply interrupt it with precisely predictable outcomes?

Still unconvinced? Consider the following: Two separate genetic loci are responsible for expressing COX enzymes. COX-1 and COX-2 are constitutively expressed in a number of organ systems, from the developing fetal brain, to the spinal cord, to the stomach and intestines, to the kidneys. The COX-2 enzyme is also triggered by an insult or damage to the physiology, and is responsible for producing inflammatory compounds that facilitate cell-to-cell signaling. If we unduly inhibit COX-1, we end up with more fatalities than are caused by AIDS, and more hospitalizations than our society can tolerate. And this is a simple, linear process that lends itself to a silver bullet? That kind of reductionist thinking ignores the wonderful, indeed infinite, complexity of the body, which is why we advocate, wherever possible, using infinitely complex herbal formulations.

How many different chemicals, polyphenols and phytonutrients are there in a blend of turmeric, green tea, *hu zhang*, rosemary, barberry, holy basil, Chinese goldthread, *Scuttelaria* and ginger? How many interactions and synergies, how many suppressions and augmentations of effects? The human mind cannot fathom. One of our great teachers and sources of inspiration, Dr. John Christopher, teaches that an herbalist is blessed with accomplishment if he or she can in one lifetime understand the constituents and workings of even *one* herb. With all respect to our admired teacher, we think even *that* is impossible. The interactions *within*, and then among, healing herbs are dynamic, non-linear and ultimately beyond our complete comprehension—which is fine, for we use those herbs to respond to medical conditions that are equally dynamic and rich in texture.

To deny the body's infinite dynamic processes is to paint humans as stationary stick figures. Silver bullets intersect with motionless lines in one place, and the result is predictable. But silver bullets pierce three-dimensional flowing, moving bodies in infinite ways. Certainly we need those bullets, sometimes, but it seems wise first to invoke more subtle, complex interventions.

BACK TO ROSEMARY . . .

Rosemary is one of nature's little dynamic miracles, a fragrant, flavorful bundle of infinite chemical complexity. In addition to the impressive properties of rosemary discussed above, what else do we know? Researchers at the Pfeiffer AM Nestle Research Center in Lausanne, Switzerland, reported in 1998 that rosemary demonstrates marked anti-tumor effects and can induce the body's protective detoxification enzymes up to four times. Japanese researchers in 1995 also reported that powerful anti-oxidants in rosemary—known as rosmanol and epirosmanol—"were shown to be effective to protect biological systems against oxidative stress." Even though it takes us somewhat off point, we can't resist reporting that researchers at the University of London, King's College, disclosed in 1996 that low concentrations of rosemary extract and its constituent carnosol had an ability to inhibit HIV infection. This conclusion was confirmed by researchers at the University of North Carolina-Chapel Hill, who reported in 1998 that derivatives of oleanolic and ursolic acid, both contained in rosemary, demonstrated potent anti-HIV activity.

Due to the multiple activities of rosemary, and the fact that several of its constituents have already demonstrated COX-2 inhibition, immune system enhancement and antimutagenic properties, we recommend that extracts of the whole rosemary leaf be used. As the research at Rutgers confirmed, the power of the whole leaf surpassed the power, albeit significant, of individual constituents like carnosol or ursolic acid. The extracts should obviously represent as much of the total phenolic activity of rosemary as possible.

Remember: The inflammatory COX-2 enzyme is encoded within our DNA and manifests throughout the body. Its imbalances can ravage multiple organ systems and lead to disability, dementia and death. When you stalk such a complex enemy with its infinite number of visible and invisible manifestations, it is good to use an equally infinite weapon. This is the glory of a broad-spectrum extract of a complex phytonutrient like rosemary.

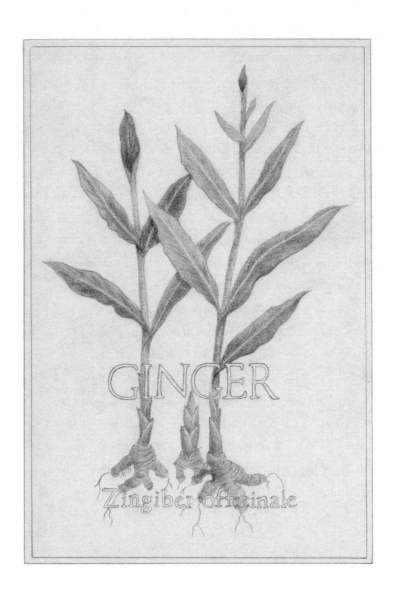

GINGER

Zingiber officinale

CHAPTER FOURTEEN

Ginger
ZINGIBER OFFICINALIS

Round amongst them [the righteous in Paradise]
are passed vessels of silver and goblets made of glass
. . . a cup, the admixture of which is ginger.
—*Koran 76:15-17*

Ginger inhibits COX-2. We state that up front, and will examine that in much more detail in a moment. But first, let us briefly consider ginger's role in the history of medicine.

An ancient Indian proverb declares: "Every good quality is contained in ginger." It is referred to in the Ayurvedic medical system as *vishwabhesaj*, the universal medicine. Confucius wrote that he was never without ginger when he ate; the surgeon general for emperors Claudius and Nero used ginger for stomach relief; and it was praised in the famous *De Material Medica* in 77 C.E.

for its ability to "warm and soften the stomach." In Japan, ginger has traditionally been used for spinal and joint pains; in the Philippines it was used for headache relief; the Chinese used it to counter toothache and hangovers; and ginger was used in Brazil, The Sudan and Papua-New Guinea to treat arthritis.

Why has ginger been revered for thousands of years, in cultures worldwide, as the most profound of healing herbs? What is THE ingredient in this pungent rhizome that has led literally billions of people to plant it, consume it, hoard it, fight wars for it and demand it for myriad medical conditions? The answer is simple: no one knows. Nor is it likely that human intelligence can ever fully fathom ginger's activities. Surely, you say, there must be one special ingredient in ginger that stands out. We respond that modern science has studied this herb for decades and has located to date at least 477 constituents, some of which, on their own, have been the subject of thousands of scientific studies.

GINGER'S CONSTITUENTS AND ACTIONS

We depart from normal form here, and ask you to be interactive with this book. Here is a challenge: Do you have the stamina to read the next ten or so pages? On these pages we have identified all the presently known (at least by us!) constituents of ginger, compiled from the monumental works of Dr. James Duke, Dr. Norman Farnsworth and our own extensive research from international medical databases. This will be an extremely difficult read, and the information is not easy to assimilate. In fact, it would take a lifetime of study to begin to fathom the interplay of the constituents, a study that we are merely in the process of performing. The purpose of this exercise will become clear, but do not think that you can or need to understand all the detail. Just read the list that follows and experience the process . . . trust us. An explanation will follow.

1. ACETALADEHYDE
2. 2-HEPTYL ACETATE
3. 2-NONYL ACETATE
4. ALPHA-FENCHYL ACETATE
5. ACETIC-ACID
6. ACETONE
7. ALANINE
8. ALBUMIN
9. ALLO-AROMADENDRENE
10. ALLO-AROMADENDRINE
11. ALUMINUM
12. GAMMA-AMINOBUTYRIC-ACID
13. ALPHA-AMORPHENE
14. GAMMA-AMORPHENE

15. ANGELICOIDENOL-2-O- BETA-D-GLUCOPYRANOSIDE
16. ARGININE
17. AROMADENDRENE
18. AROMADENDRIN
19. ASCORBIC-ACID
20. ASH
21. ASPARAGINE
22. ASPARTIC-ACID
23. BENZALDE HYDE
24. 3-PHENYL BENZALDE HYDE
25. 4-PHENYL BENZALDEHYDE
26. ALPHA-BERCAMOTENE
27. TRANS-ALPHA-BERGAMOTENE
28. BISABOLENE
29. ALPHA-BISABOLENE
30. BETA-BISABOLENE
31. CIS-GAMMA-BISABOLENE
32. BETA-BISABOLOL
33. BORNEOL
34. D-BORNEOL
35. BORNEOL ACETATE
36. (+)-BORNEOL
37. 5 ISO-BORNEOL
38. BORNYL-ACETATE
39. BORON
40. BETA-BOURBONENE
41. BUTANAL
42. 2-MENTHYLBUTANAL
43 3-METHYLBUTANAL
44 4-METHYLBUTANAL
45. 2-BUTANOL
46. SEC-BUTANOL
47. TERT-BUTANOL
48. 2-METHYL-BUT-3-EN-2-OL
49. N-BUTYRALDE HYDE
50. ALPHA-CADINENE
51. DELTA-CADINENE
52. GAMMA-CADINENE
53. ALPHA-CADINOL
54. 10-ALPHA-CADINOL
55. CAFFEIC-ACID
56. CALAMENENE
57. CALCIUM
58. CAMPHENE

59. CAMPHENE-HYDRATE
60. CYCLOCOPACAMPHENE
61. CAMPHOR
62. CAPRIC-ACID
63. CAPRYLIC-ACID
64. CAPSAICIN
65. CARBOHYDRATES
66. CAR-3-ENE
67. DELTA-3-CARENE
68. CARVOTANACETONE
69. BETA-CAROTENE
70. CARYOPHYLLENE
71. CARYOPHYLLENE OXIDE
72. BETA-CARYOPHYLLENE
73. CEDOROL
74. CHAVICOL
75. CHLOROGENIC-ACID
76. CHROMIUM
77. CINEOL
78. 1,4-CINEOLE
79. 1,8-CINEOLE:
80. 2-HYDROXY-1,8-CINEOL
81. CITRAL
82. CITRONELLAL
83. CITRONELLOL
84. CITRONELLYL-ACETATE
85. COBALT
86. CUBEBOL
87. CUMINYL ALCOHOL
88. DOCO8ANE
89. EICOSANE
90. HENICOSANE
91. TRICOSANE
92. COPAENE
93. ALPHA-COPAENE
94. COPPER
95. P-COUMARIC-ACID
96. CRYPTONE
97. CUMENE
98. CUPARENE
99. ALPHA-CURCUMENE
100. (+)-ALPHA-CURCUMENE
101. AR-CURCUMENE
102. BETA-CURCUMENE
103. CURCUMIN

104. HEXAHYDROCURCUMIN
105. DEMETHYL-HEXAHYDRO-CURCUMIN
106. CYCLOSATIVENE
107. P-CYMENE
108. P-CYMEN-8-OL
109. CYSTEINE
110. CYSTINE
111. DECANAL
112. N-DECANAL
113. UNDECANAL
114. DODECANE
115. HEPTADE CANE
116. HEXADECANE
117. NONADECANE
118. OCTADECANE
119. PENTADECANE
120. TETRADECANE
121. TRIDECANE
122. UNDECANE
123. 3-6-EPOXY-1-(4-HYDROXY-3- METHOXY-
     PHENYL) DECA-3-5-DIENE
124. 3(R)-5(S)-DIACETOXY-1-(2-4-DI-METHOXY-
     PHENYL) DECANE
125. 3(R)-5(8)-DIACETOXY-1-(4-
     HYDROXY-3-METHOXY-PHENYL)DECANE
126. 3(R)-ACETOXY-5(S)-HYDROXY- 1-
     (4-HYDROXY-3-METHOXY- PHENYL)
127. 5(8)-3(R)-DIHYDROXY-1-(4-
     HYDROXY-3-METHOXY-PHENYL) DECANE
128. 5(S)-ACETOXY-3(R)-HYDROXY- 1-
     (4-HYDROXY-3-METHOXY-PHENYL) DECANE
129. DECYLALDEHYDE
130. 6-DEHYDROGINGERDIONE
131. 6,10-DEHYDROGINGERDIONE
132. 10-DEHYDROGINGERDIONE
133. 6-DIHYDROGINGERDIONE
134. DELPHINIDIN
135. DIETHYL-SULFIDE
136. DODECANOIC-ACID
137. BETA-ELEMENE
138. ELEMOL
139. BETA-ELEMENE
140. DELTA-ELEMENE
141. GAMMA-ELEMENE
142. ELEMOL

143. ESSENTIAL OIL
144. 10-EPIZONARENE
145. 8-BETA-17-EPOXY-LABD- TRANS-
12-ENE-15,16-D IAL
146. ETHYL-ACETATE
147. ETHYL-MYRISTATE
148. ALPHA-EUDESMOL
149. BETA-EUDESMOL
150. GAMMA-EUDESMOL
151. METHYL-ETRER-ISO-EUGENOL
152. FARNESAL
153. FARNESENE
154. ALPHA-FARNESENE
155. TRANS-ALPHA-FARNESENE
156. BETA-FARNESENE
157. TRANS-BETA-FARNESENE
158. FARNESOL
159. FIBER
160. FLUORIDE
161. FLUORINE
162. FRUCTOSE
163. FURANOGERMENONE
164. FURFURAL
165. GADOLEIC-ACID
166. GALANOLACTONE
167. GERANIAL
168. CIS-GERANIC-ACID
169. TRANS-GERANIC-ACID
170. GERANIOL
171. GERANIOL ACETATE
172. GERANYL-ACETATE
173. GERMACRENE B
174. GERMACRENE D
175. GERMANIUM
176. GINGEDIACETATE
178. 4-GINGEDIACETATE
179. 6-GINGEDIAGETATE
180. 4-GINGEDIOL
181. 6-GINGEDIOL
182. 6-GINGEDIOL-ACETATE
183. 6-G-GEDIOL-ACETATE- METHYL-ETHER
184. 6-GINGEDIOL-DIACETATE
185. 6-GINGEDIOL-DIAGETATE-METYYL-ETHER
186. 6-GINGEDIOL-METHYL-ETHER
187. 8-GINGEDIOL

188. 10-GINGEDIOL
189. 4-GINGERDIONE
190. 6-GINGERDIONE
191. 8-GINGERDIONE
192. 10-GINGERDIONE
193. 6-10-GINGERDIONE
194. GINGERENONE-A
195. GINGERENONE-B
196. GINGERENONE-C
197. GINGERGLYCOLIPID-A
198. GINGERGLYCOLIPID-B
199. GINGERGLYCOLIPID-C
200. GINGEROL
201. 3-GINGEROL
202. 4-GINGEROL
203. 5-GINGEROL
204. 6-GINGEROL
205. (+)-6-GINGEROL
206. (8)(+)-6-GINGEROL
207. 6-GINGEROL-METHYL
208. 7-GINGEROL
209. 8-GINGEROL
210. 8-GINGEROL-METHYL 9-GINGEROL
211. 10-GINGEROL
212. 10-GINGEROL-METHYL
213. 12-GINGEROL
214. 12-GINGEROL-METHYL
215. 14-GINGEROL
216. 16-GINGEROL
217. DIHYDRO-GINGEROL
218. GINGEROL-METHYL
219. GINGEROL-METHYL-ETHER
220. GINGERONE
221. 6-GINGESULFONIC ACID
222. GLANOLACTONE
223. GLANOLACTONE GLOBULIN
224. GLUCOSE
225. GLUTAMIC-ACID
226. GLUTELIN
227. GLYCINE
228. GLYOXAL
229. METHOXY GLYOXAL
230. GUAIOL
231. 6-METHYL-HEPT-5-EN-2-OL
232. 6-METHYL-HEPT-5-EN-2-ONE

233. HEPTAN-2-OL
234. HEPTAN-2-ONE
235. HEPTANE
236. N-HEPTANE
237. 2-24-TRIMETHYL-HEPTANE
238. 3(S)-5(S)-DIACETOXY-1-(4'-HYDROXY-3'-5'-DIMETHOXY-PHENYL)-7-(4"-HYDROXY-3"-METHOXY-PHENYL HEPTANE
239. 3(8)-5(8)-DIHYDROXY-1-(4'-HYDROXY-3'-5'-DIMETHOXY-PHENYL)-7-(4"-HYDROXY-3"-METHOXY-PHENYL) HEPTANE
240. 3-5-DIACETOXY-1-(4-HYDROXY-3-METHOXY-PHENYL) HEPTANE
241. 3-5-DIACETOXY-1-7-BIS-(4- HYDROXY-3-METHOXY-PHENYL) MESO-HEPTANE
242. 1-7-BIS-(4-HYDROXY-3- METHOXY-PHENYL) HEPTANE- 3(8)-DIOL
243. METHYL-HEPTENONE
244. 2-HEPTANONE
245. HEXANAL
246. 2-HEXANONE
247. HEXAN-1-AL
248. HEXAN-1-OL
249. HEXANOL
250. CIS-HEXAN-3-OL
251. TRANS-HEXENAL
252. BETA-HIMACHALENE
253. HISTIDINE
254. HUMULENE
255. F-HYDROXYBENZOIC-ACID
256. 1-(4-HYDROXY-3-METHOXY PHENYL)-3,5-OCTANEDIOL
257. 1-(4-HYDROXY-3-METHOXY PHENYL)-3,5-DIACETOXYOCTANE
258. BETA-IONONE
259. IR ON
260. ISOEUCENOL-METHYL-ETHER
261. ISOGINGERENONE-B
262. ISOLEUCINE
263. ISOFUEGOL
264. ISOVALERALDEHYDE
265. JUNIPER CAMPHOR
266. KAEMPFEROL
267. KILOCALORIES
268. LAURIC-ACID

269. LECITHIN
270. LEUCINE
271. ISOLEUCINE
272. LIMONENE
273. LINALOOL
274. LINALOOL OXIDE
275. TRANS-LINALOOL-OXIDE
276. LINALYL ACETATE
277. LINOLEIC-ACID
278. ALPHA-LINOLENIC-ACID
279. LYSINE
280. MAGNESIUM
281. MANGANESE
282. MELATONIN
283. 2-METHYL-BUT-3-EN-2-OL
284. CIS-P-MENTH-2-EN-l-OL
285. TRANS-P-MENTH-2-EN-1-OL
286. P-MENTHA-1-5-DIEN-7-OL
287. P-MENTHA-2-8-DIEN-1-OL
288. P-MENTHAL-1-5-DIEN-8-OL
289. MENTHOL-ACETATE
290. P-METHA-1-S-DIEN-7-OL
291. METHIONINE
292. METHYL-ACETATE
293. METHYL CAPRYLATE
294. 6-METHYLGINGEDIACETATE
295. 6-METHYLGINGEDIOL
296. METHYL-GLYOXAL
297. METHYL-I SOBUTYL-KETONE
298. METHYL-NONYL-KETONE
299. METHYL-6-SHOGAOL
300. METHYL-8-SHOGAOL
301. METHYL-10-SHOGAOL
302. MUFA
303. ALPHA-MUUROLENE
304. GAMMA-MUUROLENE
305. MYRCENE
306. BETA-MYRCE NE
307. MYRICETIN
308. MYRISTIC-ACID
309. MYRTENAL
310. ALPHA-NEGINATENE
311. NEOISOPULEGOL
312. NERAL
313. NEROL

314. NEROL OXIDE
315. NEROLIDOL
316. 9-OXO-NEROLIDOL
317. TRANS-NEROLIDOL
318. NIACIN
319. NICKEL
320. NITROGEN
321. NONANAL
322. NONANE
323. N-NONANE
324. A-NONANONE
325. N-NONANONE
326. NONYL-ALDE HYDE
327. NONAN-2-OL
328. N-NONANOL
329. 2-NONANONE
330. CIS-OCIMENE
331. 2-6-DIMETHYL OCTA-2-6-DIENE-1-8-DIOL
332. 2-6-DIMETHYL OCTA-3-7-DIENE-1-6-DIOL
333. OCTANAL
334. 1-OCTANAL
335. OCTANE
336. N-OCTANE
337. 2-OCTANOL
338. N-OCTANOL
339. TRANS-OCTEN-2-AL
340. OLEIC-ACID
341. OXALIC-ACID
342. 9-OXO-NEROLIDOL
343. PALMITIC-ACID
344. PALMITOLE IC-ACID
345. PANTOTHENIC-ACID
346. PARADOL
347. 4-PARADOL
348. 6-PARADOL
349. PATCHOULI-ALCOHOL
350. PENTANAL
351. PENTAN-2-OL
352. 4-METHYL-2-PENTANONE
353. PENTOSANS
354. PERILLEN
355. PERILLENE
356. PHELLANDRAL
357. ALPHA-PHELLANDRENE
358. BETA-PHELLANDRENE

359. (+)-BETA-PHELLANDRENE
360. PHENYLALANINE
361. PHOSPHATIDIC-ACID
362. PHOSPHORUS
363. PHYTOSTEROLS
364. ALPHA-PINENE
365. BETA-PINENE
366. PIPECOLIC-ACID
367. POTASSIUM
368. PROLAMINE
369. PROLINE
370. PROPANOL
371. N-PROPANOL
372. PROPIONALDEHYDE
373. PROTEIN
374. NEO-ISO-PULEGOLE
375. PUFA
376. QUERCETIN
377. RAFFINOSE
378. RIBOFLAVIN
379. ROSEFURAN
380. SABINENE
381. CIS-SABINENE HYDRATE
382. SELENIUM
383. CIS-SELINEN-4-OL
384. ALPHA-SELINENE
385. BETA-SELINENE
386. GAMMA-SELINENE
387. SELINA-4, 11-DIENE
388. SELINA-3, 11-DIENE
389. SELINA-3(7), 11-DIENE
390. SERINE
391. CIS-SESQUISABINENE-HYDRATE
392. SESQUIPHELLANDRENE
393. BETA-SESQUIPHELLANDRENE
394. BETA-SESQUIFHELLANDROL
395. CIS-BETA-SESQUIPHELLAN DROL
396. TRANS-BETA-SESQUIPHEL-LANDROL
397. CIS-SESQUISABINENE-HYDRATE
398. SESQUITERPENE ALCOHOL
399. SESQUITERPENE HYDROCARBON
400. SFA
401. SHIKIMIC-ACID
402. SHOGAOL
403. 4-SHOGAOL

404. 6-SHOGAOL
405. CIS-6-SHOGAOL
406. 6-METHYL-SHOGAOL
407. ANTI-METHYL-6-SHOGAOL
408. SYN-METHYL-6-SHOGAOL
409. TRAN-6-SHOGOAL
410. 8-SHOGAOL
411. CIS-8-SHOCAOL
412. 8-METHYL-SHOGAOL
413. ANTI-METHYL-8-SHOCAOL
414. SYN-METHYL-8-SHOGAOL
415. TRAN-8-SHOGAOL
416. 10-SHOGAOL
417. CIS-10-SHOCAOL
418. ANTI-METHYL-10-SHOCAOL
419. SYN-METHYL-10-SHOGAOL
420. TRANS-10-SHOGAOL
421. CIS-12-SHOGAOL
422. THAN 8-12-SHOGAOL
423. SILICON
424. BETA-SITOSTEROL
425. SODIUM
426. STARCH
427. STEARIC-ACID
428. ALPHA-P-DIMETHYL STYRENE
429. SUCROSE
430. DIETHYL-SULFIDE
431. ETHYL-I SOPROPYL-SULFIDE
432. METHYL-ALLYL-SULFIDE
433. 1-5-TERPINE HYDRATE
434. TERPINEN-4-OL
435. ALPHA-TERPINENE
436. GAMMA-TERPINENE
437. 4-TERPINEOL
438. ALPHA-TERPINEOL
439. TERPINOLENE
440. TERPINOLENE EPOXIDE
441. ALPHA-TERPINYL ACETATE
442. THIAMIN
443. THREONINE
444. ALPHA-THUJENE
445. SESQUITHUJENE
446. BETA-THUJONE
447. TIN
448. TOLUENE

449. TRICYCLENE
450. 2,2,4-TRIMETHYL-HEPTANE
451. TRYPTOPHAN
452. TYROSINE
453. UNDECAN-2-OL
454. AN-UNDECANONE
455. N-UNDECANONE
456. UNDECAN-2-ONE
457. VALERALDEHYDE
458. VALINE
459. VANILLIC-ACID
460. VANILLIN
461. VIT-B6
462. WATER
463. XANTHORRHIZOL
464. ALPHA-YLANGENE
465. BETA-YLANGENE
466. ZINGERONE
467. ZINGIBAIN
468. ZINC
469. ZINGIBERENE
470. ALPHA-ZINGIBERENE
471. BETA-ZINGIBERENE
472. ZINGIBERENOL
473. ZINGIBERINE
474. ZINGIBEROL
475. ZINGIBERONE
476. ZONARENE
477. ZT

Overwhelming, isn't it? Does it change your perspective of what it means to drink a glass of real ginger tonic or to take a ginger supplement? If you didn't skip ahead, and if you actually read all the constituent references, you probably feel like you've run the Boston Marathon, but there was method to this madness. The weighty task of reading the ginger constituent list is to demonstrate that **ginger is the opposite of Celebrex.**

Celebrex has one molecule, designed to do one thing. Ginger has, at today's count, approximately five hundred identified compounds, many with known biological activities, working in complementary fashion to cause profound biological benefit. Each compound has some effect, whether influencing a particular enzyme or protein, or buttressing the activity of other compounds.

Take a deep breath. Ginger has multiple constituents that inhibit COX-2 and inhibit the 5-lipoxygenase metabolism of arachidonic acid, and thus deprive prostate cancer cells of their fuel for growth. Ginger inhibits the creation of prostaglandin PGE2, which has strong anti-pyretic (or anti-heat) producing effects. It balances production of inflammatory prostaglandins PGE3 and PG12, which also regulate the production of compounds that dilate the arteries. Ginger's constituents safely restore healthy platelet function by inhibiting the formation of an eicosanoid group called thromboxanes (perhaps the principal reason why people take aspirin). Ginger reduces prostaglandins that sensitize pain receptors at nerve endings, thereby demonstrating powerful analgesic (or pain-reducing) effects; has significant anti-ulcer effects compared to multiple prescription medications; contains melatonin that regulates the circadian rhythms of the body and thus stimulates both activity and sleep. As a whole, the herb has 180 times more protein-digesting enzymes than the legendary papaya, and so on. This is

117

the majesty of an herb, and this is the clearest possible illustration of how the traditional herbal approach differs from today's fashion of designer drugs.

This conceit that we can always improve the designs of nature *is* nothing more than a fashion, which is not to say that modern science has not made giant strides in the pharmacological treatment of many diseases. But, it is a tragedy that some scientists feel that we must find synthetic substitutes for the wisdom of nature. Perhaps we need to remember the words of Hippocrates, the Western world's most legendary physician, who said that we should let our medicine be our food, and our food be our medicine.

THE COX-2 STORY, WITH GINGER

We could have anticipated that ginger contains powerful COX-2 inhibitors, for it has long been recognized that ginger has significant inhibitory effects on inflammatory eicosanoids. For example, different scientific studies reflect that a therapeutic dosage of ginger demonstrates up to a 56% inhibition of inflammatory prostaglandins. The creation of these inflammatory prostaglandins appears to be mainly a function of COX-2 activity.

As even more direct proof of ginger's COX-2 inhibiting capability, recall that ginger (also *Scutellaria* and feverfew—see Chapter Twelve and Chapter Seventeen respectively) contains melatonin. This well-known hormone is also secreted by the human pineal gland, and is metabolically related to serotonin. Fascinating, isn't it, that our brain and the ginger plant (along with rice and other plant species) express the same hormone? What is also fascinating is that melatonin is structurally related to an internationally recognized NSAID known as indomethacin, and Japanese research from the 1980s confirmed that ginger has at least four prostaglandin inhibitors more powerful than indomethacin. The connections are marvelously complex.

It is now understood that melatonin regulates the human body's circadian rhythms. Not surprisingly, melatonin is used as a hormone supplement by persons wishing to facilitate sleep. Here is an interesting, and to date unexplained, connection: We know that COX-2 is expressed in nerve tissue and in the brain. So, melatonin is normally produced in the brain; COX-2 is normally produced in the brain. Any relationship? Well, as research in 1999 confirmed, melatonin exerts potent anti-inflammatory effects *via* COX-2 inhibition. These two compounds found in the brain are thus engaged in some form of complex and probably "inverse" relationship, which frankly is not at all understood. What we do know is that melatonin is yet another of the approximately five hundred compounds in ginger that is a proven, potent

COX-2 inhibitor.

We also know, and as explained in Chapter Ten's consideration of turmeric, that curcumin is a proven inhibitor of COX-2, and from the list of ginger's constituents we see that ginger contains curcumin. We thus have another source of ginger's COX-2 inhibition. In addition, research from the National University of Taiwan published in 1999 reported that a compound known as kaempferol was also "a markedly active inhibitor" of COX-2. By referring to the above list of ginger's constituents, note that kaempferol is constituent number 267.

Simply locating specific COX-2 inhibiting constituents within ginger perhaps misses the real ginger story. Frankly, in light of the extensive research on ginger's anti-inflammatory effects, it is only a matter of time before many more of ginger's plentiful compounds are confirmed as powerful and selective COX-2 inhibitors.

How can we be so confident? Logic compels the conclusion. If a powerfully anti-inflammatory compound *unduly* inhibits COX-1, then we would expect to find gastric distress, liver damage, ulcers, bleeding, kidney dysfunction and similar physiological impact. That is why the NSAIDS used for decades are being quickly supplanted by prescription COX-2 selective inhibitors, for those NSAIDS *unduly* disrupted the homeostatic, protective functions of COX-1, rather than focusing their effects on inhibiting COX-2 and balancing COX-1 in a safe, intelligent fashion. We know that anti-inflammatory ginger is gastroprotective, to the extent that its anti-ulcer properties are certainly comparable, if not superior, to the leading anti-ulcer pharmaceuticals. For example, pharmaceutical anti-ulcer compounds have proven generally unsuccessful in healing the serious ulcers that correspond to long-term NSAID use. Research with animals demonstrates that ginger has significant ability to address these pernicious ulcers. Indeed, according to the USDA Database of Phytonutrients, ginger has seventeen anti-ulcer phytonutrients—more than any other plant. Therefore, if ginger unduly inhibited COX-1, we would not expect to see these significant ulcer-preventative qualities. On the other hand, we also know that ginger safely inhibits COX-1 because of ginger's demonstrated and significant ability to restore healthy balance to blood platelet aggregation. **Simply put, ginger not only safely modulates COX-2, but it also safely brings balance to the COX-1 enzyme activity in a manner that is vastly superior to the synthetic NSAIDS, like aspirin.**

Hence, our comfort, confirmed directly and by inference, that ginger contains multiple selective COX-2 inhibitors, while also exhibiting the ability to safely bring balance to COX-1 enzyme processes. All of this is achieved without triggering the life-threatening side effects that come from synthetic NSAID use. As a consequence of ginger's anti-inflammatory capabilities, there is substantial clinical experience with therapeutic doses of ginger and the alleviation of arthritic conditions. Consider the research of Dr. Srivastava of Odense University in Denmark, who we refer to as the "Father of Modern Ginger Research":

One of the features of inflammation is increased oxygenation of arachidonic acid which is metabolized by two enzymic pathways—the cyclooxygenase (CO) and the 5-lipoxygenase (5-LO)—leading to the production of prostaglandins and leukotrienes respectively. Amongst the CO products, PGE2 and amongst the 5-LO products, LTB4 are considered important mediators of inflammation. More than 200 potential drugs ranging from non-steroidal anti-inflammatory drugs, corticosteroids, gold salts, disease modifying anti-rheumatic drugs, methotrexate, cyclosporine are being tested. None of the drugs has been found safe; all are known to produce from mild to serious side-effects. Ginger is described in Ayurvedic and Tibb systems of medicine to be useful in inflammation and rheumatism. In all 56 patients (28 with rheumatoid arthritis, 18 with osteoarthritis and 10 with muscular discomfort) used powdered ginger against their afflictions. Amongst the arthritis patients more than three-quarters experienced, to varying degrees, relief in pain and swelling. All the patients with muscular discomfort experienced relief in pain. None of the patients reported adverse effects during the period of ginger consumption which ranged from 3 months to 2.5 years. It is suggested that at least one of the mechanisms by which ginger shows its ameliorative effects could be related to inhibition of prostaglandin and leukotriene biosynthesis, i.e., it works as a dual inhibitor of eicosanoid biosynthesis.

THE 5-LIPOXYGENASE CONNECTION

In addition to safely inhibiting both COX-1 and COX-2 activity, ginger exerts substantial inhibiting effect on a somewhat related metabolic process, the 5-lipoxygenase (5-LO) enzyme. Like COX-2, 5-LO metabolizes arachidonic acid. Arachidonic acid is converted by 5-LO into a chemical called 5-HETE, which the *Proceedings of the National Academy of Sciences* reported, in 1999, was the indispensable fuel for prostate cancer cell growth. It has been conclusively determined that multiple constituents of ginger powerfully inhibit 5-LO. For example, researchers at a Malaysian university concluded that a constituent of ginger known as "eugenol" was a 5-LO inhibitor and possessed "potent anti-inflammatory and/or anti-rheumatic properties." In 1992, Japanese researchers determined that an additional eight constituents within the "gingerol" family are active against 5-LO. In a 1986 study, researchers reported that two more constituents of ginger, namely capsaicin and gingerdione, were "potent inhibitors of 5-HETE biosynthesis," which the study suggested "could account in part for anti-inflammatory and analgesic properties" of ginger. Another of ginger's constituents, curcumin, was confirmed in 1986 to be a "potent inhibitor of 5-HETE production." **Finally, the USDA Phytochemical Database, as of 1999, reports that ginger has more 5-lipoxygenase inhibitors than any other botanical source.** By our count, ginger contains a remarkable total of twenty-four 5-LO inhibitors.

THE 12-LIPOXYGENASE (12-LO) CONNECTION

A further enzymatic feature of ginger begs for serious study. Growing evidence mounts that constituents of ginger inhibit 12-LO, another enzyme that metabolizes arachidonic acid. Ginger, like *Scutellaria* and feverfew (as you will see), contains melatonin, a known inhibitor of 12-LO. Based on this, ginger and these other herbs would exhibit an ability to protect pancreatic tissue from cancerous activity. It should be noted that ginger's significant 5-LO inhibiting effect will *also* defend against pancreatic cancer cell growth.

As we have stated before, when you take an herb, you experience the effects of all its constituents. Ginger has COX-1 and COX-2 inhibiting properties, 5-lipoxygenase inhibiting capabilities, 12-lipoxygenase inhibiting capabilities, and is anti-ulcerative. It thus should play a fundamental role in the treatment of inflammatory conditions. To bring this point home on an individual level, consider this case study presented by Dr. K.C. Srivastava:

> After the diagnosis of rheumatoid arthritis all patients were treated with nonsteroidal anti-inflammatory drugs (NSAIDS) and some of the patients in later stages with corticosteroids and/or with gold salts. All the above management treatments only provided temporary relief . . . .Patient 1, an Asian male of fifty years of age living in Canada, was diagnosed as having rheumatoid arthritis. This patient began consumption of ginger in the first month following diagnosis by taking about fifty grams of fresh ginger daily after light cooking along with vegetables and various meats . . . . Pain and inflammation subsided after 30 days of ginger consumption. After consuming fifty grams of ginger daily for three months the subject was completely free of pain, inflammation or swelling. He has continued to perform his job as an auto mechanic without any relapses of arthritis for the last 10 years.

Finally, we offer a personal case study. One of this book's authors recently suffered through a serious episode of a bulging cervical disc and a pinched nerve. The neurological impairment was so severe that movement of the neck, left shoulder and arm was impossible. There was significant atrophy of the muscle tissue in the affected area, and the sensations in the left arm were quickly deteriorating from "sharp tingling" to alarming numbness. X-rays and an MRI confirmed the gravity of the problem, and three attentive and highly professional orthopedic surgeons recommended prompt surgery. In fact, the concern was regularly voiced that the recommended surgery needed to occur quickly, for the longer the nerve signal was blocked, the worse the odds for regaining full use of the left arm. This particular author, by the way, is left-handed.

The author's attention was, needless to say, quite focused on the matter of his condition. With this focus came a simple realization: When a nerve is pinched, it swells and becomes inflamed. Something, perhaps a physical injury, has caused the initial damage, but the body's own inflammatory responses can aggravate the problem, as increased swelling leads to further pinching, which worsens neurological impairment. The author, understanding ginger's anti-inflammatory capabilities, began an herbal treatment program that featured regular oral and topically applied dosages of super-critically expressed organic ginger. That was not the only herb taken orally, but it was in quantity, potency and frequency the dominant feature; and it was the only herb applied topically.

Three weeks after commencing the ginger supplementation, the author went in for a follow-up examination. The surgeon requested this exam to determine not *if*, but

126

when, the surgery was to be performed. After examining the patient, the orthopedic surgeon asked, somewhat in amazement, what the man had been doing for the past three weeks, as the inflammation had all but disappeared. More incredibly, the atrophied muscle tissue had begun to rapidly regenerate, the neurological impairment had disappeared, and the arm, while still a bit weak, was fully functional. Fortunately, this orthopedic specialist was open-minded and intellectually curious, for he was fascinated by the herbal approach. His conclusion: "I don't fully understand what you're doing, but keep doing it." Several weeks later, the author resumed his rock-climbing!

THE GINGER ANTI-TUMOR CONNECTION

Where there is COX-2 inhibition we have invariably observed an anti-tumor effect. Ginger is no exception. In a 1999 study, a ginger extract was found to possess "inhibitory activity toward EBV activation," which is considered a contributory factor in tumor promotion. In a 1998 study, two compounds in ginger were shown to possess "cytotoxic and antiproliferative effects" and were "associated with (leukemia) apoptotic cell death." Another 1998 study identified the ginger family of plants as containing "effective cancer-preventive agents" because of the "strikingly high frequency of inhibitory

127

activity." A 1996 study from the University Hospitals of Cleveland, Case Western Reserve University, noted that ginger was a source of "pronounced anti-oxidative and anti-inflammatory activities." The Case Western researchers determined in an animal study that the *topical* (on the surface of the skin) application of ginger inhibited tumor initiation and epidermal ornithine decarboxylase activity (a tumor growth factor). This well-publicized U.S. study provided "clear evidence that ginger extract possesses anti-skin tumor-promoting effects."

There is thus a substantial basis for the ancient claim of Ayurveda that ginger is the "universal medicine." Ginger is truly an herb for the ages.

For a more thorough discussion of the historical and current medicinal values of ginger, we refer you to *Ginger: Common Spice and Wonder Drug* (Herbal Free Press, 1996) by Paul Schulick.

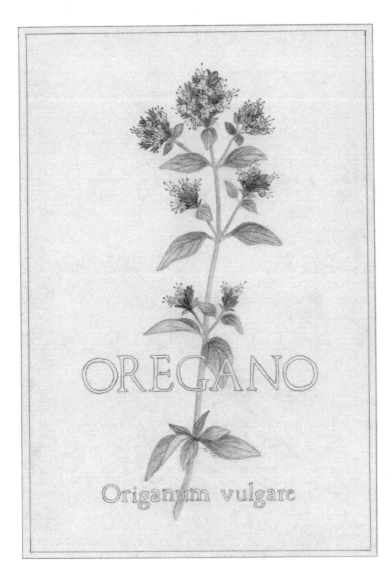

OREGANO

Origanum vulgare

CHAPTER FIFTEEN

Oregano

ORIGANUM VULGARE, LAMIACEAE

Now this is the law of the Jungle—as old and as true as the sky;
And the Wolf that shall keep it may prosper,
but the Wolf that shall break it must die....
Keep peace with the Lords of the Jungle—
the Tiger, the Panther, and Bear.
And trouble not Hathi the Silent,
and mock not the Boar in his Lair.
—Rudyard Kipling, *The Jungle Book*

We begin our discussion of oregano with this wonderful quotation from Kipling for two reasons. First, Rudyard Kipling wrote *The Jungle Book* while living in our hometown of Brattleboro, Vermont. In fact, he wrote it right down the mountain road from where we have done much of the writing of this book, and we hope that his muse has inspired us in some small way. Second, and more germane to oregano, it is one of the finest herbs for keeping "peace with the Lords of the Jungle." Inflammatory prostaglandins, leukotrienes, the COX-2 enzymes—these are the "Lords" of our body's "Jungle." We need them to police and maintain equilibrium in our body—but woe to those who antagonize them and have their ferocities misdirected. Oregano, with thirty-one known anti-inflammatories, twenty-eight antioxidants and four known potent COX-2 inhibitors, is one of the best foods to feed those jungle beasts and keep them peacefully at bay. It should be noted that with thirty-one anti-inflammatories, oregano has more recognized "peace-keepers" than any other herb in the USDA Phytochemical Database.

Oregano contains four constituent compounds that have demonstrated COX-2 inhibiting effects, all of which we have discussed in our treatment of the other herbs considered in this book: 1. apigenin (recall also green tea and rosemary); 2. kaempherol (as with ginger); 3. ursolic acid (as with rosemary and holy basil); and 4. oleanolic acid (as with rosemary). As we have previously considered these constituents in prior chapters, we will not again review their proven COX-2 inhibiting effects. What is significant about oregano, however, is that the herb has so many of the constituents in the context of a broad array of other inflammatory compounds.

One of those other anti-inflammatory compounds,

rosmarinic acid, is particularly deserving of attention. This anti-inflammatory, which not surprisingly is also presented in abundance in rosemary, has the proven capability to inhibit platelet aggregation. You will recall from Chapter Four that sticky platelets are an important factor in the spreading of cancer; we described them as sticky surfboards on which cancer cells lodged in one region could be transported to another part of the body.

Obviously a strong benefit exists in reducing platelet stickiness and thereby reducing the availability of sticky surfboards. In addition, perhaps the number one reason that people take aspirin is to reduce platelet stickiness, a means of preventing thrombotic (clotting) events like heart attack and stroke. Here is a key point to note: synthetic COX-2 inhibitors like Celebrex or Vioxx do not demonstrate the ability to reduce platelet aggregation. They reduce inflammation, but they only minimally inhibit thromboxane, the hormone that deals with the stickiness of platelets. But this inability to inhibit thromboxane is not the only bad news. Far worse, it appears that synthetic COX-2 inhibitors actually suppress a hormone that is produced in the walls of blood vessels that keeps the vessels dilated and platelets from aggregating.

We have chosen to discuss this point in the context of a chapter on oregano, but it could have been the very first chapter of this or any book on synthetic vs. natural

COX-2 inhibition. According to 1999 research from the University of Pennsylvania Medical Center that was published in the *Proceedings of the National Academy of Sciences*, the synthetic COX-2 inhibitors suppress a hormone-like substance called prostacyclin. That substance, as we just explained, is produced in the walls of blood vessels, and it both dilates or expands the vessels and helps to inhibit blood clotting and platelet aggregation. So not only do the synthetic COX-2 inhibitors do nothing to inhibit platelet aggregation via reducing thromboxane, these synthetic inhibitors actually work in the *opposite* direction and may increase the risks of clotting and aggregation.

A question must be asked: What about the natural, herbal COX-2 inhibitors—do they also inhibit prostacyclin? The answer is we don't know for sure, but let's assume that they do. What we do know from this chapter's discussion of rosmarinic acid, present in oregano and rosemary, and from this book's lengthy consideration of turmeric and ginger, is that many of these herbal COX-2 inhibitors also powerfully inhibit thromboxane, thus actively inhibiting platelet aggregation. In other words, and as we have consistently explained, these complex herbs contain natural checks and balances. Yes, they inhibit the inflammatory effects of COX-2, but at the same time they also *reduce* platelet aggregation. This is the genius of nature, and it puts into very sharp focus the potential dangers of a silver-bullet approach that only inhibits one specific enzyme.

Ironically, the scientists at the University of Pennsylvania Medical Center cautioned people to protect themselves from certain potentially dangerous side effects by taking aspirin in addition to the synthetic COX-2 inhibitors. Of course, this puts us right back in the aspirin fires again! So, it is a remarkable feature of oregano, along with ginger, turmeric and others of the herbs discussed here, that not only do they inhibit COX-2, but they also inhibit platelet aggregation. They provide the best of all worlds: a natural complex of ingredients that reduces inflammation while also providing balance to platelet aggregation. We have emphasized this critical point before, but it bears repeating: **Synthetically inhibiting COX-2 does nothing for platelet stickiness, so synthetic COX-2 inhibitors do not fully replace NSAIDS, like aspirin. On the other hand, "comprehensiveness" is the middle name of each of the featured herbs. They are, as we have explained, multi-tasking. Therefore, taking an herb like oregano reduces inflammation, reduces platelet stickiness, and does not cause bleeding or ulcers.**

Another interesting feature of oregano, and its constituent rosmarinic acid in particular, is the ability of that constituent to pass through the skin and go directly into the bloodstream and body. This transdermal capability will be considered in much more detail in Chapter Twenty-Two, but for now consider a fascinating 1989 report from the University of Cincinnati Medical Center. Researchers there properly characterized rosmarinic acid as a nonsteroidal anti-inflammatory agent (a natural NSAID), and this anti-inflammatory was applied directly on the skin in an animal study. Approximately four and one-half hours after this topical application, rosmarinic acid was detected in "blood, skin, muscle and bone tissue." Such a transdermal application of anti-inflammatories thus offers an interesting way to deliver healing constituents directly to an inflamed or diseased area, and it is a practice that has been followed in traditional medicine for thousands of years.

A Note on Extraction

It is beneficial for many reasons to separate or "extract" plant phytochemicals from the surrounding fibers and bulk of the plant. So extracted, the phytochemicals are more easily digested and utilized, and because the extraction can concentrate the phytochemicals, it is usually easier to consume a therapeutic dose in an extract form. Extracts, especially if done by competent laboratories using quality herbs, are more expensive, but they are usually the preferred form of taking an herb. By the way, an extract can be as simple as steeping a leaf (like green tea) in hot water, which is a classic water extract.

The essential constituents of oregano can be extracted "supercritically." Without going too much into the physics of supercritical extraction, it is interesting to consider this modern advance in the ancient science of herbal extraction. The supercritical extraction process uses carbon dioxide gas as the dissolving compound or solvent. We don't normally think of a gas like CO_2 as a solvent, perhaps because under normal conditions the gas does not dissolve plant constituents. But this gas behaves as a solvent when it is heated above its "critical" temperature point of 31° Centigrade and then profoundly compressed. Above that critical temperature, no amount of pressure will cause the gas to become a liquid, even if the pressure is four hundred or five hundred times normal atmospheric pressure. In that supercritical compressed condition, the gas, even though not a liquid, will behave in many ways like a fluid. It will look like a gas, but it becomes extremely dense and penetrating. This natural, non-toxic gas, compressed and deeply flowing and penetrating into the plant tissue, is capable of acting like a strong chemical solvent to extract many of the resinous, oily compounds of an herb. After the gas dissolves or draws out the resinous plant oils, the pressure is released and the gas harmlessly dissipates into the atmosphere. There is no damage to the environment, no temperature stress or damage to the plant constituents, and no chemical solvent use or residue. By avoiding chemical solvents (like commonly used solvents such as hexane and acetone), the delicate plant constituents are not corrupted or distorted either in the extraction process or in the post-extraction attempt to purge the extract of the chemicals. This extraordinary method of extraction is only available for certain herbal constituents (the lipophilic or oily plant resins of herbs like ginger, rosemary, St. John's wort, and others), and excellent supercritical extracts have been achieved for those lipophilic constituents within oregano.

Now, back to the past.

Oregano was a favorite of the early Greek physicians, who gave it its name, which means "joy of the mountain" (from *oros*, mountain, and *ganos*, joy.) The herb has delighted traditional doctors (and fine chefs) for thousands of years, and it is gratifying that modern science has confirmed the phenomenal COX-2 inhibiting, antioxidant and anti-inflammatory breath of this botanical. We recommend using this herb to keep the peace with the Lords of the Jungle. And besides, it tastes wonderful.

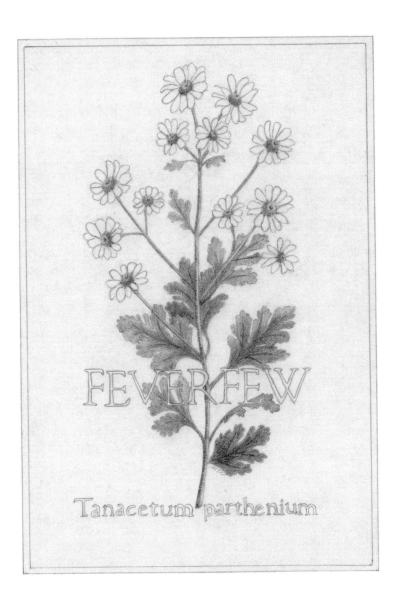

FEVERFEW

Tanacetum parthenium

CHAPTER SIXTEEN

Feverfew

ASTERACEAE, TANACETUM PARTHENIUM

Unsteady legs, untested wings:
Go fly and hear the note She sings.
She sings of ponds, of lakes, of dew,
Of marigolds and feverfew,
Of wind on wings, of life anew.
Trust Her voice to lead you true.
Trust Her, do as She has done.
Follow song to cloud and sun:
What you see, you become.
—*Becoming*, Anonymous

We advance our discussion of herbal COX-2 inhibitors with a small *hommage* to feverfew, *Tanacetum parthenium*. The name feverfew is thought to be a play on the word "febrifuge," and is precisely what its name implies: a tonic for fevers and pain. Such a traditional use, consistent with COX-2 inhibiting capabilities, was the subject of a scientific study done deep in the twentieth century—all the way back to 1996. This research by the Biomedical Research

Center of Louisiana State University was one of the first investigations into herbal COX-2 inhibitors. These scientists discovered what traditional use already demonstrated— feverfew inhibited the inflammation process. What the scientists added to our knowledge was, however, highly significant. They found that feverfew worked by inhibiting the COX-2 enzyme.

Feverfew, known also as *Tanacetum parthenium*, also contained a lactone or chemical compound called parthenolide. The action of parthenolide is somewhat complicated, but for those scientists among you, it contains a variant of the methylene-gamma-lactone, or MGL. The researchers concluded that this lactone interacted with human white blood cells called macrophages in a way to suppress a critical protein process, and this suppression in turn inhibited COX-2 expression.

Voila! This lovely little feverfew plant, with multiple daisy-like yellow flowers, can master the mighty COX-2 enzyme process. We are sure that the people of the English countryside, who have long used teas made from this herb for fevers and depression, will be pleased to know their feverfew has been decorated in this battle against inflammation.

It is also interesting to note, which was not observed by the scientific researchers, that feverfew (with ginger and *Scutellaria*) is one of nature's richest botanical sources of melatonin. As we are aware, melatonin is also an inhibitor of the COX-2 enzyme process. In addition, 1999 research from the University of Reading, UK, notes that feverfew also contains "surprisingly present" amounts of apigenin. Apigenin, you may recall, is a COX-2 inhibiting plant flavonoid present in rosemary and German chamomile, so feverfew achieves its anti-inflammatory mission from multiple chemical directions.

One of these anti-inflammatory directions in feverfew is its verified effect as an "anti-thrombotic," which means that it, like ginger and other herbs considered in this book, works to inhibit blood platelet aggregation. Since, as we've noted previously, this platelet aggregation inhibition happens to be the number one reason why millions of people take aspirin every day (to help prevent heart attack and stroke), these herbs have a wide range of benefits, without triggering the undesirable side effects. We have also explained how platelet aggregation is a significant factor in cancer metastasis, so again the ability to reduce the stickiness of the blood is welcome.

The 1999 research from the University of Reading is significant in one other respect. The scientists there were comparing the plant constituents of feverfew and *T. vulgaris* (commonly known as "tansy"), which is related to feverfew in Asteraceae species. The scientists noted that the flavonoids in both plants were dominated by apigenin, and

143

that these plant flavonoids "inhibited the arachidonate metabolism." The researchers also reported that the feverfew flavonoids were more active "as inhibitors of cyclooxygenase and 5-lipoxygenase." Thus we learn that this herb not only contains at least three proven inhibitors of COX-2, but it also inhibits the related 5-LO inflammatory enzyme that we have from time-to-time discussed in this book, most particularly with respect to cancers of the prostate and breast tissues.

Finally, and as something of a segue to the chapters to come, feverfew enjoys a well-deserved reputation as a migraine preventative. An unusual double-blind study at the London Migraine Clinic confirmed feverfew's migraine-preventing capabilities. The subjects of the experiments were people who had all previously reported significant migraine relief from feverfew. To test whether the feverfew had actual effect as distinct from placebo benefit, many of the test subjects were given a placebo that had no feverfew in it. To the great dismay of the placebo group, a substantial number of them had recurrence of migraines, and two patients had recurrence of such severity that they had to drop out of the experiment. When these patients resumed use of feverfew, their migraines again went into remission.

One note of importance regarding extraction is that some indication exists that the parthenolide constituent is not stable (which means it breaks down and basically disappears) in a dry, powered form of the feverfew extract. A resinous, supercritical extract provides a more stable form of this important constituent.

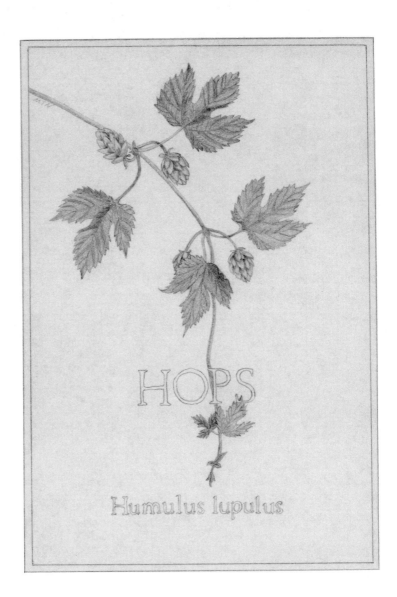

HOPS

Humulus lupulus

CHAPTER SEVENTEEN

Hops

CANNIBINACEAE, HUMULUS LUPULUS

> In the afternoon they came unto a land
> In which it seemed always afternoon.
> All round the coast the languid air did swoon,
> Breathing like one who hath a weary dream....
>
> Branches they bore of that enchanted stem,
> Laden with flower and fruit, whereof they gave
> To each, but whoso did receive of them,
> And taste, to him the gushing of the wave....
> —*The Lotos-Eaters*, Tennyson

The languor, the ease, the sleepy comfort of that mysterious land . . . so often we have wondered about the actual herb that was given to those mythic travelers. Tennyson, of course, entitled his poem *The Lotos-Eaters*, but we think a better case could be made that the "enchanted stem" could have been *Humulus lupulus*, the cousin to the marijuana plant, which people for hundreds of years have referred to as hops. Yes, the very same hops that flavor beer and ale. And no, the hop doesn't contain the psychotropic substance present in its more infamous cousin. Perhaps those legendary voyagers tasted "the gushing of the wave" in a draft of hops-flavored ale, and lapsed into their reveries . . . .

Hops: what an inapt name. The ripened cone—or strobiles—of the female hop have legendary soporific, sedating properties, and they are often combined with herbs like valerian and chamomile to calm an anxious person into comforting sleep. They have quite the opposite effect of hopping, but that name came from the old English term for climbing, which is the growing habit of this lovely vine.

But that was a digression. Now for the real late-breaking news! Based on research published on January 14, 2000, from the Department of Biochemistry, The University of Tokushima, School of Medicine, Japan, a hops constituent called "humulone" demonstrates significant COX-2 inhibiting effects. The researchers reported that humolone, which is a hops bitter, inhibited the body's re-absorption of bone, which in itself would be significant for people concerned with diminishing bone density, bone loss and damaged arthritic joints. What is more, humulone

blocked the cyclooxygenase-2 expression mediated by NFkappaB and NF-IL6.... The catalytic activity of cyclooxygenase-2 was inhibited by humulon[c] with an IC(50) of as high as 1.6 muM. These results showed that humulon[e] suppressed cyclooxygenase-2 induction at the step of transcription.

The herb's confirmed ability to inhibit COX-2, strengthen bones and promote a state of mental peacefulness perhaps explains the enormous traditional popularity of this plant. There is evidence that French and German brewers introduced the use of hops in the ninth and tenth centuries. Brewers in The Netherlands began to use hops as a flavoring in the fourteenth century, with British brewers following two centuries later. Many countries claim to be the home of the herb, but hops were used in ancient Rome, were grown throughout Britain and Europe, and are now widely cultivated in the Pacific Northwest of the United States. Traditional uses included stuffing a pillow with warm hops to allay anxieties and induce sleep. Teas of hops and either chamomile flowers or poppy heads were used, according to British herbalist Mrs. M. Grieve, "for swelling of a painful nature inflammation [and] neuralgic and rheumatic pains . . . ." Mrs. Grieve observed that such a tea "removes pain and allays inflammation in a very short time." As an earlier chapter noted, chamomile contains a COX-2 inhibitor called apigenin, and poppy heads contain, well . . . you know.

To add modern notes to the healing reputation of this herb, researchers at Oregon State University determined in 1999 that flavonoids in hops were potential chemopreventatives against breast and ovarian cancer. Researchers in Japan also determined in 1998 that humulone inhibited the growth of monoblastic leukemia cells.

If an herb has given relief for centuries, if not millennia, we must respect it. It has proven its worth in the most important laboratory of all, the laboratory of human experience. Hops deserve our appreciation, not only because they are now recognized COX-2 inhibitors, but because they also help the body prevent cancers and induce a state of emotional comfort and mental peace. Those are precious qualities today, and they come from the feminine fruits of such a graceful, climbing herb.

We began this chapter with a somewhat whimsical theory that Tennyson's travelers may have stumbled upon the "enchanted stems" of the hops plant. But *The Lotos-Eaters* is just a poem, and our speculation is just that. What we know for certain, however, is that there is a magnificent herb that eases pain and inflammation and induces sleep. It is, therefore, something to consider in the evening hours, perhaps with chamomile and another stress-reducing COX-2 inhibitor, holy basil.

Let us end, therefore, with another thought from Tennyson, as he neared the end of his life. He wrote to his grandson of his years at Locksley Hall:

> Forward, backward, backward, forward, in the immeasurable sea.
> Swayed by vaster ebbs and flows that can be known to you or
> me.

A lullaby of sorts, these lines remind us of the complex currents that move our lives. Those currents course through our bodies, as well, and that is why the *Humulus lupulus*, whose very name is something of a lullaby, is so welcome for the nighttime relief it offers.

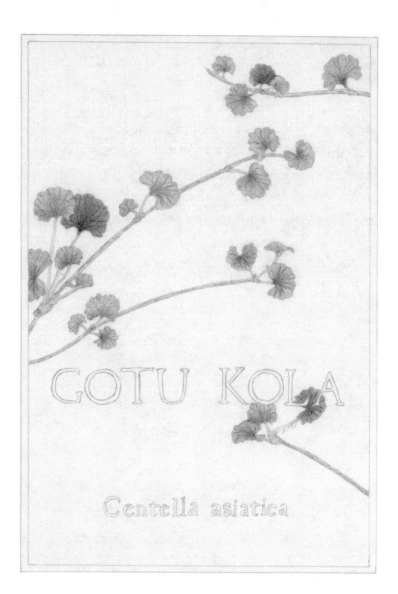

GOTU KOLA

Centella asiatica

CHAPTER EIGHTEEN

COX-2 *Inhibition* *and Alzheimer's Disease*

For weykness of ye brayne. Against weyknesse of the brayne and
coldenesse thereof, sethe rosemaria in wyne and lete the
pacyent receye the smoke at his nose and keep his heed warme.
—From the *Grete Herbal*, quoted in Grieve, *A Modern Herbal*

There's rosemary; that's for remembrance. Pray, love, remember...
—Ophelia, in *Hamlet*, Act IV, Scene V

Yes, there is rosemary for remembrance. Rosemary, rich in ursolic and carnosic acids, is a potent COX-2 inhibitor, and there is now compelling evidence that COX-2 inhibitors reduce brain inflammation and thus reduce the ravages of Alzheimer's disease (AD). But, long before we knew of COX-2 and its natural chemical suppressors, Shakespeare wrote of rosemary and remembrance. It turns out that the bard's neighbor was none other than noted sixteenth century herbalist John Gerard,

153

who wrote in 1597 that, "Rosemary comforteth the braine, the memorie, the inward senses." Let's find out why.

Much like the connection between chronic NSAID use and reduced incidence of colon cancer, researchers have long observed an association between chronic NSAID use and a reduction in the incidence and severity of Alzheimer's disease. Scientists at the University of British Columbia reported in 1998, "Twenty epidemiological studies . . . published to date indicate that populations taking anti-inflammatory drugs have a significantly reduced prevalence of Alzheimer Disease or a slower mental decline." Researchers from LSU Medical Center in New Orleans recently put it quite plainly: "Long-term treatment by nonsteroidal anti-inflammatory drugs has been shown to decrease the incidence of Alzheimer's Disease." The researchers explained, in far more complex terms, that "Individual hypervariability in COX-2 RNA message abundance may reflect various degrees of expression of [AD]-related inflammatory processes." In layman's terms, an inflamed brain, over-expressing COX-2, is more prone to Alzheimer's disease.

Alzheimer's disease is sadly quite pervasive, striking approximately 10% of the population over the age of sixty-five; 20% over the age of seventy-five; and increasing by an additional 10% over each additional decade of life. It diminishes the lives of millions of our precious and beloved family members and friends, and it is a threat to each of us. There are risk factors that can be somewhat managed, such as avoiding head trauma wherever possible, but the reality is that Alzheimer's disease can strike anyone. We live in a society where brains are inflamed, literally on fire, from the heat of COX-2 processes.

BRAIN PLAQUE

A closer look at our most current understanding of this disease reveals a remarkable connection between Alzheimer's disease and other inflammatory conditions. First, we know that the brains of patients with Alzheimer's disease show, in specific regions, the accumulation of plaque comprised of beta-amyloid (Abeta) peptides. This is not as complicated as it may sound. The brain, for reasons not yet clear, just gets gummed up, much like other parts of the body can build up plaque deposits that cause trouble. It appears that an enzyme in the brain "snips" or grooms protein strands that are out of place, and the snipped molecules accumulate to form the Abeta plaque.

By comparing the Abeta plaque to other plaque formations in the body, we are not suggesting that these plaques are made of the same molecular "stuff." Yet, just as with the plaque in atherosclerotic arteries or the plaque on teeth, the Abeta plaque materials are not functional, can become inflamed or cause inflammation, and can

155

result in disease. The similarity exists among various plaques that they themselves are generally not the real medical problem. The medical challenge is presented by the complications that can result from the body's inappropriate, confused response to plaque (tooth decay, gum disease, stroke and heart attacks).

Where there is hardening of the arteries there is arterial plaque. Similarly, where there is Alzheimer's disease there is *always* Abeta plaque. But, we can extend this comparison of body plaques in the other direction as well. People can have dental plaque *without* developing gingivitis; can have arterial plaque without getting a stroke; and can have brain Abeta plaque without developing Alzheimer's disease. In fact, many people with such brain plaque never develop, or do not fully develop, Alzheimer's disease.

It is literally critical to understand why some people have brain plaque but do not suffer from Alzheimer's disease, and two recent studies cast important light on this issue. In one of the studies, conducted at Washington University in St. Louis, Missouri, (the *alma mater* of both authors of this book) researchers at the School of Medicine did a long-term study of twenty-one healthy elderly subjects (average age at the time of death 84.5 years). Nine of the twenty-one subjects had "strikingly high plaque densities" in an important region of the brain. Two of those nine died of head injury before any sign of cognitive impairment. The other seven demonstrated "very mild cognitive impairment." The remaining twelve subjects demonstrated no cognitive impairment and "had few or no neocortical lesions." The researchers concluded that "senile plaques may not be part of normal aging but instead represent presymptomatic or unrecognized early symptomatic Alzheimer's Disease." In other words, the researchers considered the plaque to be abnormal, and an early indicator of the onset of Alzheimer's disease. To these researchers, it seemed only a matter of time before the plaque led to the cognitive impairment associated with this disease.

As for the second study, two years after the Washington University research a fascinating article was published in the journal *Neurology*. It offered a slightly different perspective on senile plaque. While not contradictory to the earlier Washington University research, this subsequent study pointed to some contrasting conclusions. Researchers from British Columbia noted that anti-inflammatory drugs had often been suggested as a possible treatment for Alzheimer's disease. To test that concept, they autopsied brain tissue. They compared "postmortem brain tissue from elderly, nondemented, arthritic patients with a history of chronic nonsteroidal anti-inflammatory drug (NSAID) use . . . and nondemented control subjects with no history of arthritis or other condition that might promote the regular use of NSAIDS . . . ." The two groups studied, then, were: people with no Alzheimer's disease who were not on NSAIDS, and people with no Alzheimer's disease who were on NSAIDS. These scientists wanted to see what effect the use of anti-inflammatory drugs had on physical conditions that might correlate with Alzheimer's disease, and the results were remarkable.

In both the NSAID-treated group and the control group, 59% of the subjects had some senile plaque. Note: none of the subjects demonstrated *any* dementia or other expression of Alzheimer's disease, but the *majority* of them had senile plaque. There was no difference between the two groups of subjects in the number or types of senile plaque, or the maturity or nature of the plaque. Moreover, the degree of neurofibrillary pathology (we'll return to that concept of twisted, curly and tangled brain fibers in a moment) was similar in the two groups. Was there any difference? Yes—the control group (those who had not been taking any anti-inflammatory drugs) had almost three times the number of activated microglia as the NSAID-treated group. Activated microglia are part of the inflammatory-response mechanism within the brain. When the microglia are activated, there is going to be an inflammatory response. Think of fire and smoke: activated microglia are fire, inflammation is smoke. They go together, like disease and fever. The authors concluded that if anti-inflammatory drugs work to reduce the severity or avoid the onset of Alzheimer's disease, it is through suppression of the inflammation response, not through inhibiting Abeta plaque deposits.

What do we conclude from these two important studies? First, that the presence of senile plaque, the Abeta deposits, does not in and of itself mean that a person has any degree of Alzheimer's disease or is likely to develop the disease. Indeed, the British Columbia study revealed that 59% of non-demented subjects had varying degrees of senile plaque at death, and even the Washington University study simply opined that the plaque deposits "may" not represent normal aging, but may be presymptomatic of Alzheimer's disease. Second, others and we conclude that the Abeta plaque on its own does not cause dementia, but somehow triggers a fire of inflammation in the brain that can be avoided or reduced by anti-inflammatory agents. This is a profoundly important concept since all of us—authors and readers of this book alike—may well have numerous deposits of senile plaque, although we pray that none of us has any manifestation of senility. Certainly there is the potential irritant, but there is not yet any irritation.

Even though the image of plaque deposits in the brain is disturbing, keep in mind that most of us can live with this plaque, for decades, without it diminishing our mental functioning. (For most of our lives brain plaque may be like having dental plaque without cavities or gingivitis.) Unfortunately, however, inflamed plaque catches up with some millions of us as we turn sixty, seventy or eighty. But, the converse is also true that, for millions of other elderly, the plaque simply never gets inflamed to the point that it is problematic. The issue is whether we as individuals can do anything to improve our odds.

It goes without saying that inhibiting the formation of the Abeta brain plaque would be the obvious first strategy. Just as the best strategy for avoiding gingivitis is proper oral hygiene to prevent the build up of dental plaque, and the best strategy for avoiding atherosclerosis is proper diet and antioxidant support, the best strategy for avoiding Alzheimer's disease is avoiding the formation of senile plaque. The problem is, we don't know exactly what *causes* it to form, other than that it is constructed of the Abeta peptide. But, there is fascinating historical confirmation that inhibiting the formation of this brain plaque works to promote mental clarity.

In the ancient herbal medical tradition of Ayurveda, an herb called *gotu kola*, of the species *Centella asiatica*, has been used with great success, for thousands of years, to promote mental clarity and brain functioning in the elderly. The herb has legendary efficacy as an anti-inflammatory and to relieve mental fatigue, and the mere fact that it has continued to be used by millions of people over the millennia is strong evidence that it works.

Some fast facts on *gotu kola*: It is indigenous to India and the southern United States. It grows best in marshy areas and riverbanks. It is one of nature's richest sources of the chemical asiatic acid. Asiatic acid, in turn, is a demonstrated inhibitor of Abeta plaque formation. As you would say at the end of a geometry proof: QED, that is, the thing is proven! *Gotu kola* has worked for thousands of years to promote mental clarity, and it inhibits Abeta brain plaque. We thus have comfort that the strategy of inhibiting the formation of brain plaque is wise to pursue, and we also have the comfort of knowing that a particular herb has performed this task with revered distinction. Clearly, therefore, the intelligent use of an extract of *gotu kola* should be one of the first lines of defense against Alzheimer's disease.

The Alzheimer's-*gotu kola* connection illustrates one of the great values of ethnobotany and traditional medicine. Those sciences can confirm from the successful experiences of millions of patients over thousands of years that a compound is beneficial and safe. In contrast, modern medicine is by nature confined to extremely short-term tests with a limited population of subjects. This is not meant as a criticism of modern medicine, but to suggest that ethnobotanical experience is an invaluable resource for today's scientists, and that it can suggest important strategies for dealing with today's medical crises. There is great wisdom in preserving our botanical diversity around the globe, for some plant on the other side of the world may hold the key to solving a critical medical challenge for someone near and dear.

THE ONSET OF BRAIN INFLAMMATION

We established that the primary strategy is not to get Abeta senile plaque in the first place. However, for tens of millions of us it is too late for that, and all the *gotu kola* in the world may not be enough to avert the formation of that deposit for some. Environmental insults, chemical reactions, head injuries and stresses and similar affronts to the brain may trigger Abeta plaque formation, and we need to understand what to do to keep that plaque from diminishing our mental clarity.

Many of us die old and sharp. That's the goal. In the Vedic tradition of ancient India, the elderly are revered for sacred wisdom and spiritual cognition. We think wistfully of the council of elders in traditional societies, and of Justice Oliver Wendell Holmes authoring brilliant legal opinions into his nineties. On a personal level, the beloved grandmother of one of the authors, then in her nineties, was asked if she was beautiful as a young child. She responded that she was the loveliest of children, and then with a twinkle in her eye whispered "and who is there now to say that I wasn't?" Yes, subtle wit, grace and wisdom can characterize a ninety-year-old mind. The key is to age with clarity. And the key to that is to keep the Abeta plaques from getting inflamed.

If we can keep COX-2 inflammation under control in the brain, we can avoid all or much of the challenge of Alzheimer's disease. That is the essential lesson of modern neurological science. We will explain this in detail, but first an outline, a brief road map, of the incontrovertible relationships among brain inflammation, COX-2 and Alzheimer's disease.

A ROADMAP TO THE
DEVELOPMENT OF ALZHEIMER'S

Often, a person with Alzheimer's has suffered some type of head injury or trauma, whether it's from a physical event or some food or chemical "insult" to the brain. Beta amyloid (Abeta) plaque, also called senile plaque, forms in certain regions of the brain, perhaps as a consequence of the trauma or insult. There is a relationship, still not fully understood, between these plaque deposits and the existence of curly fibers and tangles in the brain. It turns out that these curly fibers and tangles are, in Alzheimer's patients, present not only in the brain but can be found also in the pancreas, ovaries, testes and thyroid. In other words, there is something knotted and tangled going on in the overall Alzheimer's physiology, not just localized in the brain. The plaque, on its own or in conjunction with the curly fibers and tangles, irritates the brain and triggers an inflammatory reaction.

The inflammatory reaction is certainly complex, but at its core is the COX-2 enzyme. COX-2 is over-expressed in the neurons of an Alzheimer's patient. The oversupply of COX-2, whether on its own or due to the metabolites it creates, makes the brain react with more toxicity to the plaque formations. In other words, a brain overstocked with COX-2 becomes overheated. As a consequence, there is clear evidence of free-radical damage inside the plaque and curly fibers of Alzheimer's patients. Their plaque gets inflamed, and oxidation byproducts (the opposite of what antioxidants do, and why you take them!) are created that damage and poison the brain. Where there is an excess of COX-2 in the brain, you will find the death of neurons, those delicate cells that carry the signals and messages in the brain.

In cases of people who have taken NSAIDS, such as aspirin, on a chronic basis for pain relief, there is a side effect of suppressing brain inflammation. The NSAIDS do not reduce the plaque deposits—they work by reducing the inflammation that results from the plaque and curly fibers that twist in the brain. With chronic NSAID use, the suppression of inflammation is achieved by the reduction in COX-2 expression in the brain, which results in less neuronal death. As a consequence of neurons being protected (or at least not killed during the inflammation response), there is a demonstrated and strong correlation between COX-2 inhibition and avoiding or reducing Alzheimer's disease.

The issue of brain inflammation is so profound in modern societies that each of the major points noted above deserves further elaboration, which follows.

Head Trauma. We start with the repeated observation that head trauma has been associated with Alzheimer's disease. This observation was recently tested in an experimental setting in a Swedish laboratory, where rats were subjected to "moderate" brain injury. After three months, the rats were tested for signs of persistent inflammation, and chemicals indicating inflammation were present in large areas of their brains. The researchers concluded that long-term inflammation following trauma seems a factor in "traumatically induced dementia."

Head trauma can result in many ways, from the obvious car and bicycle accidents to the taking of recreational drugs. One distinguished radiologist reports that, in his clinical experience, 25% of the cranial MRIs taken of members of the Baby Boomer generation reflect some degree of plaque formation, which he correlates to the pervasive drug use of that generation.

The wise course is to take appropriate, reasonable measures to protect the brain from injury or chemical insult. People should always wear seatbelts, people on bikes should always wear helmets, and it is best to avoid inhaling or consuming substances that can shock or overwhelm the brain. As parents, we also note with concern the implications of this caution regarding sports such as football, ice hockey and soccer (from "heading" the ball). The rash of concussions suffered in those sports is a serious cause of concern due to possible long-term consequences. Are competitive, contact sports valuable in numerous ways? Unquestionably. But, is it wise to engage in sports that often result in head trauma? Each parent must make a personal decision, but steps should be taken to minimize the likelihood of head trauma. This means helmets, mouth guards and other prudent safety measures.

Senile Plaque. Perhaps because of trauma or chemical insult, Abeta plaque often forms in the brain. As we explained, Abeta plaque has been found in 59% of the brains of elderly non-Alzheimer's individuals. It is, therefore, a fact of life for most of us. And given the aging of our population, Alzheimer's disease is also a fact of life for most of us, either personally or with dear ones.

Curly Fibers and Tangles. An uncomfortable image, to be sure. Fibers curl and tangle inside the brain, get inflamed, and the mind suffers. As put succinctly by Swiss researchers in 1999: "The filamentous brain lesions

166

that define Alzheimer Disease (AD) consist of senile plaque and neurofibrillary tangles." So these neurofibrillary tangles, also called curly fibers, trigger some form of inflammation and result in brain lesions. What is interesting is that these curly fibers are not localized in the brain. The Swiss researchers, studying twenty-one different tissues from twenty-four Alzheimer's disease cases, determined that the curly fibers and tangles found in the brain lesions were also present in the liver, pancreas, ovary, testes and thyroid. The researchers weren't sure just what that meant, but the observations "indicate that the formation of 'curly fibers' and 'tangles' is not unique to the central nervous system. The results suggest that Alzheimer's Disease might be a systemic disorder . . . ." In other words, there are irritants throughout the body in Alzheimer's, and one manifestation of the irritation is in the brain.

Brain Inflammation. This is the key to understanding Alzheimer's disease. It is not the plaque, not the curly fiber, but the associated inflammation that is the cause of neuronal death. In a thorough review of Alzheimer's disease published by Harvard researchers in 1998, the scientists explained that the breakthrough came in the 1980s when the Alzheimer amyloid deposits were found to contain, in addition to beta-amyloid peptides, other proteins that are normally observed during acute inflammation.

These researchers made the distinction that the Abeta plaque is the precursor to Alzheimer's disease, but not Alzheimer's disease itself. The plaque forms "amorphous deposits" that induce, in some people, an inflammatory reaction. The process works like this: The plaque and the curly fibers cause an irritation. When the brain is irritated, the cells in that region sense an assault or trauma and secrete compounds that activate alarms, or microglial cells, which in turn secrete other chemicals that signal danger. These chemical sirens, called cytokines, in turn trigger the release of yet other chemicals that interact with the amorphous plaque. This interaction causes the squishy plaque to harden into mature strands or filaments of Abeta. It's almost as if the soft and squishy plaque is viewed as an invader, and a chemical counterattack is waged to thwart the invasion. That would be fine if the inflammatory response turned itself off properly, but it doesn't. The neurons get alarmed and confused by these Abeta deposits, become tangled and die.

COX-2 and Brain Inflammation. As we have explained in this book, one of the jobs of COX-2 is to stimulate the production of inflammatory prostaglandins. To draw an analogy: When the town is attacked, the call goes out for troops. The soldiers ride in, furiously, on horseback, and sometimes they attack everything in sight that looks at all funny. Walls come down and fields get trampled in the process, but hopefully the invasion is put down and the soldiers ride away. Sometimes, however, the cavalry forgets to go away. The soldiers think that the threat persists, and they set up permanent camp. This is now a huge problem. A town can handle the noise and mess and mayhem for a short while, but if the madness continues it becomes perhaps a bigger problem than the original perceived threat.

In the United States constitution the Bill of Rights holds a law that says that civilians can't be forced to quarter the military. Unfortunately, no such natural law exists in our bodies, and the inflammation SWAT team can sometimes take over. The rules of the body change when that team is around. Those soldiers—the massive white blood cells—do their work too well, and inflammation becomes a fact of life. We have explained this process before, but it is worth revisiting.

We also learned from the earlier chapters that COX-2 is present in the brain. You may recall that one scientist from Johns Hopkins expressed uncertainty over what would happen in the brain if COX-2 was chronically inhibited by pharmaceutical agents. But, because COX-2 is naturally present (or available to be summoned) in the brain, it must have a biologically important role to play. The role it plays in the brain is the same as it

169

performs elsewhere; that is, when induced by threat, trauma or insult, it works to create the inflammatory prostaglandins, stimulate the danger signals, and call in the forces. We know this because COX-2 levels are known to increase in brain neurons after electroconvulsive stimulation (a.k.a "shock therapy"). We also know that levels of brain expression of COX-2 correspond to the density of the Abeta plaque, and that neurons in an Alzheimer-diseased brain show elevated levels of COX-2 expression.

The picture is clear. The COX-2 inflammatory response is out of balance with the actual threat, and the plaque gets inflamed. Just as with atherosclerosis, the real problem is when the arterial plaque gets inflamed and ruptures, leading to stroke and heart attacks. In the brain, the Abeta plaque gets inflamed, and that leads to a host of other problems considered below.

COX-2 Inflammation and Toxicity. Toxicity means precisely what you think. Something becomes poisonous and damaging. When the plaque becomes inflamed, and when there is an over-expression of COX-2 in the neurons, the brain becomes more susceptible to Abeta toxicity. The plaque deposits start to fester, the brain produces chemicals in response to, or as part of, that inflammation, and those chemicals are toxic. We will examine some of those toxic substances in the next chapter, but as a preview, the key is oxygen free-radical poisoning. An example of the poisoning process was demonstrated experimentally by researchers at the University of Pittsburgh in 1998. A condition known as "global ischemia," or total oxygen deprivation, was created in the brains of the rat subjects. It was as if they suffered massive strokes, which cut off oxygen to their brains. The researchers determined that COX-2 indicators increased in the rats' brains after the ischemia, or oxygen deprivation, was induced. Conversely, rats that had been treated with a COX-2 inhibitor had a higher survival rate of brain neurons after the ischemia. The researchers concluded that COX-2 activity "contributes to...neuronal death after global ischemia." Simply put, the over-expression of COX-2 correlated to brain toxicity and the death of neurons. Not a good thing, to say the least.

NSAID Use and Reduced Alzheimer's Disease. As the research from the University of Pittsburgh reflects, the use of a COX-2 inhibitor reduced the toxicity or poisonous nature of brain inflammation. COX-2 inhibition accomplishes this not by reducing the amount of senile plaque in the brain, but by suppressing the undue inflammation that can occur in response to the plaque. This is consistent with more than twenty long-term studies reflecting that persons taking anti-inflammatory drugs on a chronic basis, such as those who use anti-inflammatories for arthritis, have a significantly reduced incidence of Alzheimer's disease or a slower mental deterioration. It is logical to ask, then, *Why aren't all people taking NSAIDS to prevent or reduce the severity of Alzheimer's disease?* The answer to this is the same as for NSAID use and colon cancer. Yes, using NSAIDS reduces the incidence of Alzheimer's disease (and certain cancers), but the side effects of chronic NSAID use are worse than the cure. Remember that more people died last year from the side effects of NSAID use than from AIDS, and you get the picture. The medical establishment's enthusiasm for the pharmaceutical synthetic COX-2 inhibitors, and our enthusiasm for herbal COX-2 technology, is that it is possible to reduce inflammation without inhibiting the beneficial activities of COX-1. We believe that while there are some times and places for the pharmaceutical COX-2 approach, there is always a role for the herbal strategy to play. With respect to Alzheimer's disease it is simple—by reducing systemic inflammation on a long-term basis, evidence is overwhelming that we can reduce the incidence or severity of Alzheimer's disease.

We desire the gift, the blessing, of a long, full life. Ironically, that blessing carries a special challenge, for the brain can slowly succumb to the same inflammatory processes that the body uses to protect the brain. Each assault, each insult, to the brain triggers an inflammatory response, and the inflammatory response creates neuro-toxins that erode the long-term vitality of the mind.

We all sense that our world delivers regular insults to our precious nervous systems. Whether it's from the chemicals in our foods, improper drug use (prescription or otherwise), physical trauma to the head, or just from the weight of suffering in the world, the brain gets overwhelmed. No one has ever expressed this more powerfully, or more succinctly, than the poet William Blake who, in his masterpiece "Auguries of Innocence," wrote:

> Every outcry of the hunted Hare
> A fibre from the Brain does tear.

We hear this outcry everyday of our lives, and we hope for a balm, a remedy for the rips and tears. Thankfully, nature has placed herbs that soothe and protect in habitats across the world, and this is one of the great comforts of herbal COX-2 anti-inflammatories.

CHAPTER NINETEEN

Free-Radical Damage and Alzheimer's Disease

The famous historian of science, Thomas Kuhn, observed that scientists are always captives of the paradigm, or prevailing views, of their era. In other words, if scientists of a certain period had made an intellectual commitment to a model of science (like the earth is the center of the universe), then those scientists would only see facts that fit into or support that model or paradigm. Conversely, if a fact did not fit into a paradigm, then the scientist wouldn't see it at all, or would reject it as irrelevant. It's as though scientists wear sunglasses that filter out certain frequencies of light. Every now and then, however, an Einstein, Pasteur or Newton appears, smashes the old sunglasses, and puts on the filters of a new paradigm. Enter the Theory of

Relativity, the Germ Theory of Disease, and the Laws of Thermodynamics. Those leaps of intellectual understanding and insight change how everything is seen. At first the breakthroughs are often scorned, then they are resisted, then slowly adopted, and finally become so accepted that people feel "it has always been so."

That revolution in thought is precisely what is happening today in modern medicine with the discovery of the action of the COX-2 enzyme. Our understanding of the pivotal role of this newly discovered enzyme forces us to reevaluate our former understanding of biological processes and disease. We are forced to put on new glasses and see the body in totally different terms.

The COX-2 enzyme has always been present in humans. It is built into our genetic code, and we share that code with other organisms deep in our evolutionary history. But until this decade, we did not even know that it existed. We didn't have a paradigm, the proper pair of glasses, to even look for its existence. Once we discovered that its actions were at the core of numerous functions and diseases, we started to see evidence of COX-2 activity everywhere.

For example, in a 1999 article published in the *Journal of Clinical Endocrinology and Metabolism*, researchers from Amsterdam noted the curious fact that people with Alzheimer's disease often have disturbed sleep, night-time restlessness, and other indications that their body clock isn't functioning properly. A brain hormone called melatonin is the main hormonal messenger setting the circadian rhythm of the brain, and these researchers discovered that people with Alzheimer's disease have dramatically decreased levels of melatonin in their brain and spinal fluids. The COX-2 connection? You may recall from our review of ginger that one of its constituents, a plant form of melatonin, is a recognized COX-2 inhibitor, and its domain is in the brain. Thus, it is not at all surprising that persons with dramatically decreased levels of melatonin exhibit the chronic inflammation and elevated COX-2 levels associated with Alzheimer's disease. It is not at all surprising, but the association was neither made nor predictable prior to our current understanding of the role of elevated COX-2 expression in Alzheimer's disease.

There is another, and we feel far more profound, manifestation of COX-2 over-expression that we can only now begin to understand. As we explained in the previous chapter, where there is COX-2 over-expression in the brain there is also inflammation. It is not plaque that causes Alzheimer's disease; instead, it is *inflamed* plaque that ravages neurons. Once again, as we determine that inflammatory COX-2 lies at the core of the disease, we can predict that something is being created in the inflammation process that is killing neurons. That prediction is absolutely correct, and there is overwhelming evidence that free radicals of oxygen, thrown off in the inflammatory process, are responsible for neuronal death and brain impairment.

We need to stress that while no one knows precisely the sequence of events leading to Alzheimer's disease, we do know that there is a clear cause and effect relationship between COX-2 and inflammation. We also know that there is a clear statistical relationship among COX-2, inflammation and Alzheimer's disease. But what is it about inflamed senile plaque that ends up killing surrounding neurons? As we said in the preceding paragraph, it appears to be oxidized fat and free radicals of oxygen, thrown off in the inflammatory cascade, that poison the neurons. There are lipids [such as Omega-3 and Omega-6 polyunsaturated fatty acids, (PUFA)] and low density lipoproteins (LDL) throughout the brain. The PUFAs are used by the body to build neuronal membranes.

On the other hand, we don't know precisely why or how the LDLs get into the brain. Remember from our discussion of ginger in Chapter Fifteen that LDL gets into the arteries, is oxidized, creates foam, the foam hardens into plaque, the plaque gets inflamed, and *Voila!*, atherosclerosis, stroke and heart attacks. We learned that the enzyme lipoxygenase, like its cousin cyclooxygenase, oxidizes fats and lipids, and this oxidizing creates a by-product, namely, free radicals of oxygen. Sometimes scientists call these free radicals by another exotic name, namely, "reactive oxygen species," which simply means that this menacing species of oxygen like to react with other molecules, bind with them, steal their electrons, and generally destabilize them at every level, even at the level of their DNA. The important thing to remember here is that the body is trying to deal with LDL—it considers LDL a problem, and its enzyme forces attack it and break it down. As a consequence, free radicals of oxygen are created or released, which wreak their own special havoc. You have no doubt heard of being killed by "friendly fire." Caught in the crossfire of battle, you are undone by your comrades' bullets. This is, in a way, what is happening in the environment of the inflamed brain dealing with LDL.

In a 1999 issue of *Brain Pathology*, scientists from the University of Kentucky autopsied the brain tissue of Alzheimer's sufferers, and found that their brains showed increased levels of lipid (fat) peroxidation. Simply put, the fatty materials in their brains turned rancid, spoiled by exposure to free radicals of oxygen. Hence the term "peroxidation," or the process of oxygen interacting with the lipids. In addition, the Alzheimer's brains studied contained less PUFA, and more by-products of oxidized PUFA. It's rather obvious: cyclooxygenase (specifically COX-2) exists to oxidize fats. PUFAs are fats in neuronal membranes, and if COX-2 and lipoxygenase run rampant, those enzymes break down or oxidize the PUFAs in

179

neuronal membranes. The PUFA levels go down, the corrosive byproducts of oxidized PUFAs go up, and the brain equilibrium is destroyed.

These same scientists at the University of Kentucky also discovered that Alzheimer's brain tissue had oxidized DNA. This literally means that some DNA had literally been broken apart and rusted by the reactive oxygen species let loose by inflammation. They also found oxidative stress byproducts in neurofibrillary tangles and senile plaque, and lipid peroxidation byproducts in brain and spinal fluid. This is not a pretty picture. It was one thing to picture the brain inflamed, but another to realize that the biological consequences of that inflammation are rancid brain fats, dead neuronal tissue and degraded DNA. The conclusion reached by these researchers is absolutely on target and critical for understanding an herbal response to the problem; that is, it is necessary to address both the inflammation and the oxidative stress in an Alzheimer's brain. An effective therapy needs to treat both aspects of the problem.

In the words of Uncle Remus, "You can hide the fire, but what will you do with the smoke?" You can put out or minimize the fires of COX-2 and lipoxygenase inflammation, but what about the smoke, the oxidative cloud, which sweeps across the brain. One could take Celebrex or Vioxx, which are both, by design, powerful inhibitors of an oxidating enzyme. They are thus both, by definition, antioxidants in one sense—they inhibit one form of oxidation. But what the inflamed brain needs, we believe, is a broader, more comprehensive approach. There is, after all, that darned smoke to deal with, and we need to provide the body with as many "smoke removers" as possible. This is where traditional herbal medicine shines most brightly, for in just one herb, such as ginger, there are dozens of different free-radical scavengers that can bind with reactive oxygen species and neutralize the cloud of destruction let loose by inflammation.

For purposes of "smoke removal" we again turn to the COX-2 inhibiting botanicals, many of which are shown to have significant antioxidative effects. Frankly, traditional herbalists are bemused by the public's current sense that the antioxidants *par excellance* are synthetic compounds like ascorbic acid (vitamin C) or isolated vitamin E. Yes, those are antioxidants, and they do interact with and thus scavenge or neutralize free radicals. But to revere those simplistic compounds as the greatest antioxidants of our time would be like revering paint-by-number art as a da Vinci masterpiece. Where are the complexities, the subtle nuances, the multiple antioxidative capabilities of a ginger with up to five hundred known constituents; of green tea with over four hundred constituents; of *Scutellaria* with free-radical scavengers so powerful that they can rescue an arrested heart poisoned by reactive oxygen out of control? These, and the other herbs mentioned in the prior chapters, are champion free-radical scavengers. If they are combined in a traditional, broad-spectrum formulation a person could literally enjoy the benefits of hundreds of free-radical scavengers attacking the reactive oxygen species— the brain cloud—from multiple phytochemical directions. And, not only will these champion botanicals protect the brain from COX-2 "smoke damage." Their antioxidant capabilities also serve and protect the joints and organ systems throughout the body as they contend with the COX-2 beast. In other words, although we are highlighting these antioxidants in the context of Alzheimer's disease, it is just as appropriate to laud them for protection against other COX-2 related inflammatory conditions such as arthritis and cancer. Perhaps this is why herbal formulations from traditional medical systems often feature several herbs used in combination. Just check the many herbal constituents of sacred Ayurvedic and Chinese formulations to quickly confirm this formulation approach.

If we were asked to identify just one herbal antioxidant as a balm for the mind, it would be difficult to choose. Surely there is rosemary, "rosemary for remembrance," and to this day students in Greece burn sprigs of rosemary before examinations to stimulate their minds. There is, after all, an unquestionable mental stimulation from rubbing an extract of rosemary, in a proper lotion or oil base, upon the scalp. So is rosemary the one? No, for then you would be foregoing ginger's multiple antioxidants and green tea's legendary catechins and other polyphenols. There is also significant research supporting the efficacy of *Scutellaria*, turmeric and *hu zhang* as cerebral free-radical scavengers.

The answer is that our brain is too precious to put it in the care of just one herbal antioxidant, no matter how impressive that one might be. Your central nervous system is buffeted by so many hostile forces from within and without that it deserves the protection of a full complement of herbal antioxidants. The herbal COX-2 inhibitors described above, together with a comprehensive herbal and nutritional program, form a solid foundation for a lifetime of healthy brain functioning.

CHAPTER TWENTY

Other Phytochemical Strategies for Dealing with Brain Plaque & Related COX-2 Inflammation

The focus of this book has been on COX-2 inflammation, and that is clearly the primary condition that gives rise to Alzheimer's disease. This condition is complex, and in some respects it is more a "syndrome" than one specific disease process. There can be many imbalances or disturbances at work in creating the mental deterioration, and there are thus complementary approaches to the Alzheimer's challenge. Just as with our treatment of arthritis and cancer in this book, we do not explore the many herbal approaches to fully address these dread diseases. Rather, our principal focus has been on the means of controlling the inflammation process itself. With that in mind it is appropriate to consider four fascinating additional connections between COX-2 inflammation and Alzheimer's disease.

1. Beta-Amyloid Plaque Inhibition / Toxicity Strategy

As we have previously explained, the problem is not so much that beta-amyloid plaque exists in the brain, but that it gets inflamed and toxic via COX-2 activity. Having said that, the image of plaque deposits, amorphous or defined, snaking through the brain is not a pleasant one, and it would certainly be better if people did not have to contend with them at all. Like having a splinter in your finger—it only hurts when it gets infected and inflamed, but it's better never to get one in the first place. Or, if you happen to get one, to get it out promptly once it's there. Fortunately, there is a known antagonism between a chemical called asiatic acid and the Abeta plaque. Asiatic acid inhibits the formation of Abeta plaque, and that chemical is naturally present in *gotu kola*. No doubt this is why *gotu kola* has for perhaps thousands of years been used to promote mental clarity.

Turmeric, another of the herbs highlighted in this book, in addition to its many COX-2 inhibiting and anti-oxidant properties, has also demonstrated an ability to protect neuronal tissue in one other important respect. When the Abeta plaque becomes inflamed, it appears to throw off toxins that induce neuronal apoptosis, or the cellular suicide of brain cells. In research published in the journal *Neuroscience Research* in 1998, scientists determined that curcumin (which is present in both turmeric and ginger) has an ability to "abolish Abeta-induced apoptotic cell death."

2. Beta-Amyloid Wound Healing Strategy

Why would wound healing be of significance in Alzheimer's disease? Because the Abeta plaque can get inflamed, like the atherosclerotic plaque in arteries, like joint tissue in arthritis, and like tissues under the assault of incipient cancer. It is these open wounds in the arteries, brain, joints and other tissues that can fester, disable and kill. This is even more of a problem for the elderly, for their wound healing capabilities become compromised over time. This is not only true on a bio-chemical level, but we can confirm it in our daily lives. The sprained ankle that healed in a day when we were young might linger for weeks when we get older. A skin wound heals quickly and well in the young (hence greater scarring with the young, for the body repairs aggressively when we are young), but a sore may take weeks to heal as we age. And those are the sores and wounds we can see *on* our bodies. How about the wounds *inside*: in the arteries, in the joint tissue, in areas attacked by cancer and in the brain? They simply don't heal as quickly or as thoroughly, and that protracted festering is a serious health concern.

Anything that safely promotes wound healing,

wherever those wounds are in the body, is therefore especially prized for the elderly. In this regard, consider *gotu kola*'s many capabilities. First, the asiaticoside from *gotu kola* stimulates collagen formation. Collagen is a protein that is the main component of connective tissue (like cartilage in the joints), and indispensable in certain wound healing processes. Second, a topical application of asiaticoside twice daily for seven days was found, in a laboratory setting, to cause an increase in both enzymatic and non-enzymatic antioxidants in newly formed tissue. This increased antioxidant activity was significant: 35% increase in superoxide dismutase (SOD), 67% in catalase, 49% in glutathione peroxidase, 77% in vitamin E and 36% in ascorbic acid. These are wonderful wound healing factors, and the topical application of asiaticoside derived from *gotu kola* also corresponded to decreased problematic substances, such as a 69% decrease in lipid peroxidation (rancid fat) levels.

A good first line of defense, therefore, is to avoid or minimize plaque formation before it triggers a COX-2 reaction and free-radical damage. A good second line of defense is to heal the wound should it arise. *Gotu kola* works effectively on both defensive fronts. As *gotu kola* is a revered Ayurvedic herb, it seems only appropriate to quote an Indian sage who lived untold centuries ago, Rishi Patanjali. His fundamental instruction in life was *heyam dukam anangatam,* or "avert the danger before it comes." That's perfect advice in life and great advice with respect to inflamed brain plaque.

3. The Curious Nitric Oxide Strategy: A Case for *Brahmi*

You may recall from the cancer model in Chapter Four that there is an evanescent chemical wisp called nitric oxide that flits about the body at speeds almost too fast to measure. The 1998 Nobel Prize for Medicine was awarded to three pharmacologists who discovered it, like an atomic trace in a cloud chamber, dashing about the body. These decorated scientists concluded that nitric oxide plays a role in a number of bodily functions, including the regulation of brain activity. Nitric oxide is thought to facilitate the maturing of thought into action, but frankly no one knows precisely what it does or how it works. Let's call it a "messenger molecule," and leave it at that. Scientists do theorize that nitric-oxide imbalances are unhealthy and likely to be at the root of many disease conditions. Nitric oxide is thought to spike at points of inflammation.

Again, the nitric oxide situation is a question of balance, as it has been for every other process we have examined. We must have the compound; nitric oxide appears to be everywhere and nowhere at once; and certain herbs are suspected to stimulate or balance its activity in a positive way. One such herb is *brahmi*, also known as *Bacopa monnieri*, and it has been used as a neurotonic for over three thousand years in the Ayurvedic tradition of India.

Brahmi, indigenous to India, is an amphibious plant living on lakeshores and the banks of slow flowing rivers. Its principal traditional use has been as a tonic for mental exhaustion and forgetfulness. A paste made from its leaves was also used to treat joint pain, and it is used in Ayurvedic formulations for stress and anxiety.

Brahmi contains two identified active constituents called Bacosides A and B. Research conducted almost forty years ago at the Central Drug Research Institute of India determined that the Bacosides stimulated protein synthesis and thereby improved memory and learning. Dr. Robert Furchgott of the State University of New York, one of the three Nobel laureates responsible for the discovery of nitric oxide in the body, tested *brahmi* in his laboratory and determined that "this compound appears to release Nitric oxide . . . ."

Modern science is inching its way to an understanding of nitric oxide and *brahmi*, but three thousand years of its successful use as a mental tonic encourage us that it belongs in our apothecary for healthy brain functioning.

4. Cerebral Thrombosis / Berberine Strategy

As we have previously discussed, one of the inflammatory hormones created by cyclooxygenase out of arachidonic acid is a compound called thromboxane. Thromboxane promotes the blood platelet stickiness" that we have identified as a factor in the metastasis of cancer cells. Chinese researchers in 1995 concluded that berberine, a constituent of barberry and Chinese goldthread, had the ability to inhibit the formation of thromboxane and therefore was protective of the brain in conditions of cerebral ischemia. (Recall that cerebral ischemia is the situation in which the brain is deprived of oxygen, such as in a stroke.) Berberine has the ability to keep the blood unsticky, and not clotting, and is therefore protective of brain tissue when it is so challenged.

It has been fascinating for us to discover the pivotal role COX-2 inflammation plays in the Alzheimer's disease process. Once we understand the relationship between COX-2 inflammatory processes, the creation of toxic free radicals and other neurotoxins, and the disease itself, we could then see how that brain inflammation was so closely related to inflammatory processes involved in cancer and arthritis. It is reassuring to intellectually understand that taking an herbal COX-2 inhibitor because you have inflamed joints has the supremely wonderful side effect of also protecting tissues from cancer metastasis and protecting the brain from neuronal death. The fact is that the synthetic COX-2 inhibitors will, over time, demonstrate some of these interconnected benefits, but it would be impossible for any one synthetic compound to offer the range of anti-inflammatory benefits that time-tested botanicals have been scientifically shown to provide.

CHAPTER TWENTY-ONE

Omega-3: A Complement to Herbal Inhibition of Inflammatory COX-2

I must down to the seas again,
for the call of the running tide
Is a wild call and a clear call
That may not be denied.
—*Sea Fever*, John Masefield

We passionately agree with the poet John Masefield: the call to the sea, and the essential Omega-3 nutrients that it plentifully yields, may not be denied. Perhaps one reason we are drawn to the ocean, that it plays so on our imaginations when we are separated from it, is that the ocean is saturated with the minerals and amino acids that comprise our bodies. Indeed, many scientists believe that eons ago the volcanic warmth and electricity of the earth triggered a reaction between the atmosphere and the chemically-rich ocean that gave rise to the first simple

193

amino acids.

We may never know precisely how earth's complex, carbon-based life forms (like us!) got their start, but think of the life biomass within the ocean now. Untold myriad life forms, immeasurable quantities of microalgae, plankton and deep water fish. These are the true treasures of the deep—and so much of that biomass is a crucial source of Omega-3 fatty acids with which we build our cell membranes and create the hormones that regulate the "tides" of our existence. We thus turn our attention now, as we near the end of this book, to the gifts of the sea, for as Rachel Carson expressed so simply fifty years ago in her masterpiece *The Sea Around Us*, "For all at last return to the sea."

Certain fatty acids are an indispensable part of our diet. Indeed, one of the fatty acids (alpha-linolenic acid) is called "essential" because it, and other Omega-3 fatty acids that are derived from it, are simply critical to life. Our bodies cannot manufacture the true essential fatty acids on their own. Therefore, in the case of alpha-linolenic fatty acid, we must either eat foods containing it or containing Omega-3 fatty acids derived from it such as docosahexaenoic acid (DHA). Let us emphasize that without this essential fatty acid or its Omega-3 derivatives we would physically struggle and possibly die. Forget everything you have ever thought you knew about how "bad" all fats are—it is a heresy that must be debunked.

When we eat the essential and other fatty acids, we incorporate them into our cell membranes. If we eat the correct fatty acids, our cellular membranes are strong, flexible, and discriminating. One part of the fatty acid chain loves water, one part loathes it. One form of the fatty acids, the *cis*-fat form, has an arrangement of hydrogen atoms that make the molecules bend and flex in just the perfect way to build smoothly functioning cell walls. Once we build the cell walls from these fatty acids, they are like the perfect children's sack lunch for school. Not only do we metabolize what's *within* the lunch bag (the nutrients inside the cells), but our enzymes (like COX-2 and the lipoxygenases) can metabolize the fatty acids *in* the membranes.

When these enzymes interact with the fatty acids, we create eicosanoidal hormones like the prostaglandins we have spoken of. Some of these prostaglandins are inflammatory; others are anti-inflammatory. Some thicken the blood, some reduce platelet aggregation thereby thinning the blood. A majestic system of hormonal checks and balances is built on and out of the fatty acids.

As is obvious, we need these prostaglandins and other eicosanoids, even the extremely inflammatory ones created by COX-2. When they are present in balance with our bodies and our environments, they sustain life.

Without the fatty acids, we cannot manufacture these hormones. So, with respect to fat consumption, our teenage children might say "live with it." We certainly can't live without it.

Our focus here is on the fats that heal by taming any unbalanced and raging COX-2 inflammation. Let's review a few key facts on fatty acids, particularly the Omega-3 series.

What are the Fatty Acids? Fatty acids are a particular class of carbon chain molecules, with an organic acid group at one end (which contains a certain weak acid that loves and binds with water) and a carbon-hydrogen fatty chain at the other (which hates and repels water). Imagine a cat hating water on the same leash with a dog loving water! Our cells use this "split personality" to create phospholipid membranes that selectively attract and repel water. Our bodies cannot manufacture all of the fatty acids we must have for life, and those are called the essential fatty acids. From those essential fatty acids the body can assemble other derivative fatty acids that actually make their way into the membranes. Arachidonic acid, one of the stars (and sometimes the villain) of the COX-2 story, is technically *not* an essential fatty acid because we can both obtain it from meats and manufacture it from another true essential fatty acid, which is a fatty acid called linoleic acid. How do we manufacture it? Here's a short biochemistry lesson: The body first converts linoleic acid (an essential one) to gamma-linolenic acid, next to dihomo-gamma-linoleic acid, and then finally to arachidonic acid. Arachidonic acid is an Omega-6 fatty acid. This creation of arachidonic acid is a deliberate and usually slow process, but if we eat a diet rich in meats we are consuming "prefab" arachidonic acid. As we shall explore later, that is usually a poor idea.

Double Bonds. Now for some quick chemistry facts. (You will not be quizzed! In fact, you can skip this paragraph if chemistry bored you in school, but in any event no straining is required—it is all just a preface to the important conclusions to follow.) The fatty acids contain a chain of carbon atoms (we are carbon-based life forms), one after another, with sometimes sixteen, eighteen, twenty or more carbon atoms creating the chain. Arachidonic acid, for example, with which COX-2 interacts to create inflammatory hormones, has twenty carbon atoms in its chain. The carbon atoms, for mystical or quantum mechanical reasons that we will not consider, need to fill their outer electron orbit in order to achieve a stable, complete form. To gain that quantum balance, the carbon atoms can share electrons with hydrogen or other atoms, or they can bond with themselves. When they bond with themselves, it is called a double bond. If the fatty acids do not *ever* double bond, and if *all* the bonding opportunities are saturated with hydrogen electrons, then the resulting fat is "saturated." Conversely, if a double carbon bond exists, the fat molecule is not fully saturated with hydrogen, and is thus "unsaturated." The first time a carbon double bond appears in an unsaturated fatty acid determines the fat's Omega number. So, when the first double bond appears on carbon 3 or 4, counted from the methyl end, then the fat is an Omega-3 fatty acid. If the first carbon bond is at the sixth carbon position, counted from the methyl end, it would create an Omega-6 fatty acid. Arachidonic acid is an Omega-6 fatty acid, which by definition is unsaturated. Because arachidonic acid has multiple double bonds, it is deemed "poly" unsaturated. If a fatty acid had only one double bond, it would be "mono" unsaturated. So much for the quick chemistry primer.

As we promised, you will not be quizzed. Absorb the information to your comfort level, for it is purely background, and helps define some often misused or misunderstood terms.

The Inflammatory Prostaglandin Connection. We have considered this briefly before, but here is a quick review leading to some additional important connections between Omega-6 arachidonic acid and inflammation. Lest you get weary of this detail, trust us that it leads to an important conclusion.

Hormones called prostaglandins regulate and respond to conditions in the body. Related eicosanoids, the inflammatory leukotrienes, are created by 5-lipoxygenase.

Series 1 prostaglandins *reduce* platelet aggregation and inflammation; series 2 prostaglandins *increase* platelet aggregation (clotting factors) and inflammation; and series 1 and 3 prostaglandins basically act as a check on the production of too much series 2 inflammatory prostaglandins. These are the hormonal checks and balances.

Series 2 prostaglandins, such as PGE2, are made from the arachidonic acid stored in and released from cell membranes. PGE2 and other inflammatory hormones are created out of the interaction of COX 2 with arachidonic acid. Basically, COX-2 is oxidizing the unsaturated arachidonic acid, which by its very nature attracts oxygen. In other words, arachidonic acid exists in the body to be oxidized. In the words of the Terminator (in the movie by the same name), "It's nothing personal." It's just arachidonic acid's job.

This does not mean that we should not eat foods containing fatty acids, no more than it means we should stop breathing oxygen. We need the fatty acids, we need oxygen, and sometimes we need to oxidize the former with the latter. This is crucial—it's all in the balance.

On the other hand, we do not need to breathe polluted or toxic air, and we do not need to eat burned, toxic or "trans" fats. Those should be consistently avoided, as they pose serious health challenges.

The key is that there are only so many places in the body for fatty acids—only so many membrane job opportunities to fill, as it were. Many membranes, such as those in the brain, prefer to use or incorporate Omega-3 fatty acids (not an arachidonic acid) over the Omega-6 series from which arachidonic acid is made. Moreover, in conditions of inflammation, the Omega-3 series competes with arachidonic acid for enzyme metabolism, and the metabolites of Omega-3 are not as inflammatory or vexatious as the arachidonic acid metabolites.

This last point is so critical that we suggest you read it over enough to get the full impact. Omega-3 fatty acids, like DHA, compete with Omega-6 arachidonic acid for a location in cell membranes and compete for the enzymes that metabolize fat. The oxidized metabolites that ultimately come out of the Omega-3 series, which are free radicals of oxygen, are less inflammatory and less biologically active than the metabolites of arachidonic acid.

Armed with this knowledge, we control our own inflammation destinies. If we want to have:

- flexible, healthy cell membranes
- fat that burns clean, like a high grade of fuel

- fat metabolites that are less inflammatory and carcinogenic,

then we show a dietary preference for the Omega-3 fatty acids and we consume the proper herbal antioxidants that manage or eliminate the excess free radicals that inevitably arise from time to time. Really, this is the sum and substance of the COX-2 story. And it is not difficult. The herbal antioxidants we need, otherwise described in this book as herbal COX-2 inhibitors, are available, as are excellent sources of Omega-3 fatty acids, particularly the DHA form that we prefer.

If our diet has a proper ratio of Omega-6 to Omega-3 fatty acids (which should be in the range of 2:1 to 4:1, not the 10:1 to 40:1 ratios that modern Western diets present); and if there is an abundance of high quality DHA together with the proper herbal anti-inflammatory support; then we should expect to experience less injurious, less severe and more "balanced" COX-2 inflammation. Again, the goal is not to eliminate all inflammation all the time. That would be unnatural, and would deprive the body of the oxidative weapons it needs for a strong immune defense. The goal is for measured, intelligent inflammation in accord with true need and with our pain tolerances. Conversely, we seek to avoid and inhibit runaway inflammation that is out of control and causing more harm and suffering than good. Such injurious inflammation, for example, as that which cripples, supports the growth of cancers or disables the mind.

If we have a good, unspoiled, solvent-free and not over-heated form of Omega-3 fatty acid (not the dreaded rancid, smelly cod-liver oil of memory) we should expect to have less arthritic inflammation and a stronger antioxidant profile. For example, researchers at a university hospital in The Netherlands reported in 1996 that the use of Omega-3 fatty acids induced improvements in rheumatoid arthritis, psoriasis and colitis, and that pro-inflammatory cytokines decreased. This is precisely what we would expect from our analysis of the COX-2 inflammatory cascade.

Researchers in the Department of Rheumatology at Albany Medical College, New York, also reported in 1996 that investigations from Europe, the United States and Australia "described consistent improvement in tender joint scores" with Omega-3 supplementation. This report, in a journal aptly named *Lipids*, went on to explain that some patients with rheumatoid arthritis are able to discontinue nonsteroidal anti-inflammatory drugs when they are given Omega-3 fatty acids. In short, "A large number of peer reviewed publications from around the world have established the utility of dietary supplementation with n-3 [Omega-3] fatty acids in reducing tender joint counts and morning stiffness in patients with [rheumatoid arthritis]." Again, when Omega-3 is present to modulate the inflammatory COX-2 process, that is precisely what we would expect.

Many other observed, actual health benefits are associated with Omega-3, and particularly DHA, consumption. These actual, observed benefits are fully consistent with the COX-2 strategy and predictions of our analysis. To identify just a few:

• The Albert Einstein College of Medicine noted in the journal *Carcinogensis* in 1999 that Omega-3 fatty acids inhibit proliferation of breast cancer cells, while consumption of Omega-6 fatty acids stimulated cancer cell growth. DHA exerted more beneficial cancer inhibition than another Omega-3, EPA. On that note, our review of the scientific literature strongly suggests that if we consume DHA Omega-3, the body will "retroconvert" or create from the DHA any EPA that is required.

• In a 1995 issue of *Oncology*, Japanese medical researchers determined that DHA and EPA suppressed breast cancer cell growth and proliferation.

On the flip side, having too little or diminishing DHA in the brain is associated with cognitive decline during aging and Alzheimer's Disease. In addition, there is a strong correlation between DHA deficiency and depression. The neuronal membranes with ample DHA are clearly healthier, more supple and less inflamed, all of which support cognitive functioning and emotional balance.

A FOCUS ON DHA SUPPLEMENTATION

A plentiful supply of Omega-3 fatty acids, especially DHA, is an important part of the COX-2 inhibition program. That is the Omega-3 strategy. As we have observed throughout previous chapters, the herbal strategy is also compelling. How do they work together? Not surprisingly, they are fully complementary and augment each other's efficacy.

First, a look at conventional, allopathic medicine's take on this issue. The Department of Medicine of the University of Texas Health Science Center proposed, in 1994, that combining nonsteroidal drugs with protective Omega-3 fatty acids may provide additional protection against age-associated rise in malignancy and immune disorders. *The American Journal of Clinical Nutrition* reported in 1991 that the clinical use of anti-rheumatic drugs combined with DHA and EPA "improve[d] joint pain in patients with rheumatoid arthritis" and was beneficial with ulcerative colitis. The corollary to this is equally important: there is an observed *negative* relationship between the anti-inflammatory effectiveness of conventional NSAIDS (and the newer pharmaceutical synthetic COX-2 inhibitors such as Celebrex) and the consumption of sources of arachidonic acid. Arachidonic acid added to the diet reduces the effectiveness of these drug agents, which makes sense. This acid is the fuel of inflammation, and when it is abundantly present it works against the anti-inflammatories. As scientists from the Royal School of Medicine in London succinctly put it, "the supply of arachidonic acid to COX-2 determines the effectiveness of NSAIDS." Again, this is clear guidance. First, increase intake of Omega-3. Second, decrease arachidonic acid or its Omega-6 sources.

What is true in the world of anti-inflammatory drug activity is equally valid in the herbal approach. We strongly recommend, when using herbal COX-2 inhibitors, to increase the intake of Omega-3, particularly DHA-, fatty acids. Conversely, it is wise to reduce the intake of arachidonic acid sources.

Finally, we have explained that fatty acids exist to be oxidized. They are drawn to oxygen, they help bring oxygen into and through tissues and cells, and they are readily oxidized by various enzymes. Logic dictates that when consuming even the highly beneficial and life-supporting Omega-3 fatty acids, it is mandatory to have a well-stocked arsenal of herbal antioxidants to handle any free-radical mischief and strengthen the positive effects of the fatty acids. For example, Harvard Medical School researchers concluded in 1994 that the antioxidant curcumin (which is present in both ginger and turmeric) "in combination with dietary fatty acids" lowered the production of oxygen free radicals. Research from India, also in 1994, indicated that combining Omega-3 fatty acid with eugenol, an antioxidant constituent from cloves, augmented the anti-inflammatory effect of the fatty acid. In the researchers' opinion, "combinations of dietary lipids with spice principles like eugenol can help in lowering inflammation."

The COX-2 enzyme can be controlled, but sometimes the body gets stressed or pushed out of balance. Then, that enzyme can act like an overly eager, confused and undisciplined soldier who sometimes rushes off into battle before it is time, fires wildly even at his own troops and won't listen when the generals tell him to stop fighting. But, under the guidance of powerful and wise herbal commanders, and if fed rations of the right fatty acids, this soldier can proudly serve and defend.

BACK TO THE SEA

We thus go back to the source of life, and derive physical and mental strength from the organic oil of the ocean. We should obtain that nourishment from fresh, deep-water fish such as salmon, and we emphasize "fresh." A "fishy" smell means that the lipids, the fatty acids, have oxidized, which is a polite way of saying the fat has gone rancid. We don't ever recommend consuming pre-oxidized fat, whether it has oxidized from losing its freshness or from being fried or burned. And the fish should not be from fish farms. Those fish typically do not eat a diet of marine algae, and thus do not store the Omega-3 fatty acids that come from that natural food source.

Of course, there are Omega-3 fish oil supplements, but care should be taken to choose the highest quality fish oil products. You simply do not want to be consuming unnecessary oxidized products, so the supplements should have extremely low peroxidation levels. In addition, when you consume a beneficial fatty acid you must always keep in mind that you are consuming a fuel for free-radical formation. For that reason, we strongly recommend ingesting herbal antioxidants (like ginger and cloves, sources of researched complements curcumin and eugenol, respectively) to support the body's healthy utilization of the fatty acids. Finally, we do not believe in consuming hexane or other chemical solvents, so we recommend Omega-3 products that have not used such solvents in the extraction process. Unadulterated products as we have described are out there, but you may have to look for them!

Another attractive source of DHA is something of a modern wonder. Fish don't create Omega-3 DHA or EPA, they obtain it from algae. So could humans, and such algae-rich DHA is now commercially available. Moreover, creative farmers are feeding that algae to hens, whose eggs become suffused with the healing wonders of DHA.

We personally use those eggs, and it is a pleasure thinking of the beneficial DHA so easily obtained.

If we take advantage of these simple supplementation opportunities and return to the unbounded ocean and its nourishment, we can effect a "sea change" and restore inflammatory balance to our lives.

CHAPTER TWENTY-TWO

Alternative Delivery Systems of Herbal COX-2 Inhibitors: Transdermal Herbalism & Aromatherapy

Thou anointest my head with oil,
my cup runneth over.
—King David, *Twenty-third Psalm*

It is reasonable to believe that [the topical ginger extract] inhibited
the action of the [arachidonic-acid induced] tumor promoter....
—*Cancer Research*, March 1996,
Case Western Reserve University

We suppose you are wondering what the *Twenty-third Psalm* has to do with the inhibition of arachidonic acid induced tumors by the topical application of ginger extract. That's a fair question. We believe the answer is that the ancients, like King David, knew something that we are only now beginning to rediscover. Our ancestors knew that herbs and oils, like olive oil and ginger extracts, had powerful healing effects if applied on the skin. Such an anointing made David the king; on mammals, it prevents COX-2 arachidonic acid metabolites from causing skin tumors. Both sound like pretty good deals to us!

We do not in any way mean to trivialize the anointing of David's head with oil. In the Bible, olive oil was used for such purposes, and we now know that olive oil inhibits arachidonic acid metabolism by the 5-lipoxygenase enzyme. Later in the Bible, he who was prophesized to have his head anointed with oil was termed *mashiach*, or "messiah." *Mashiach* literally means "the one whose head is anointed [with olive oil]"—thus the term "God's Anointed One." In the ancient Greek of the New Testament, *mashiach* translated to "Christ." We therefore deeply appreciate the roots, in the Western world, of the practice of applying precious herbs and oils to the head and skin.

The only puzzlement is how these ancient sacred practices came to be viewed by some as relics of a different time. By 1697 the Oxford English Dictionary describes *unction* (the anointing with oil) as a ceremony "derived from primitive antiquity" (J. Potter); and by 1768 unction is said to have been practiced by "the primitive fathers," and is grouped with "exorcisms . . . signatures of the cross, and lustrations by holy water" (Tucker).

Maybe we read too much into these dictionary references, but we sense some condescension, a feeling that these practices are quaint, but not something for educated moderns. Somewhere along the way we became cynical. Maybe we went through the motions, but unction became a relic of the past, for the poor, superstitious "primitives." Like King David and Christ.

Nevertheless, within Christianity today these ancient uses of oil are still practiced in sacramental rituals, and anointings with sacred herbs are common in the East. You have seen pictures of the *sadhus* and *gurus* of India with their foreheads covered in a sandalwood paste. This is said to be protective, offering the enlightened the succor of a cooling herb. In the medical system of Ayurveda, the channels (*shrotas*) of elimination and energy are purified by *abhyanga*, or herbal sesame oil massage. The unsettled mind's fluctuations are calmed in Ayurveda by *shirodhara*, which is the slow, rhythmic pouring of warm herbalized sesame oil on the forehead. And the restlessness born of a *vata dosha* imbalance is abated by the rubbing of *ghee*, a clarified butter, upon the soles of the feet.

Moving from the subtle and sacred to the ridiculous and profane, there is the now humorous story of the chemist Albert Hoffman. Fifty years ago, Hoffman was experimenting with a new chemical compound, and he accidentally brushed his skin against the chemical. His

211

experience must have deeply surprised or alarmed him, for the compound was lysergic acid diethylamide (LSD), and just one accidental transdermal application was enough to send him on the world's first acid trip.

These chemical transdermal exposures can be uplifting, bizarre and sometimes gravely toxic. For example, in 1984, researchers from the Massachusetts Department of Environmental Quality Engineering determined that certain diluted and toxic chemicals could more easily enter a bather's physiology through skin absorption than from drinking the undiluted chemical. On the other hand, the pharmaceutical industry was quick to develop supposedly healthy "patches" for estrogen, for nicotine, and surely soon for this and that novel drug. The pharmaceutical industry understands that the transdermal application of drugs is a powerful delivery system. We say, what works for drugs works for herbs too—and will work particularly well with the herbs we recommend for COX-2 inhibition.

THE BIOLOGICAL CASE

Drugs and herbs enter the body through the skin; that is fact. An interesting question is why, and the answer will take you back to an earlier chapter of this book. But first, consider some basic skin physiology. The skin is the largest organ in the body. Yes, it is an organ, albeit an external one; with specific jobs to perform just like its internal co-workers. In one square inch of skin there are approximately 650 sweat glands, 100 sebaceous (oil-producing) glands, 78 heat sensors, 13 cold sensors, 165 structures that perceive pressure, 1300 nerve endings, and 19 yards of blood vessels.

And remember, all you see is the surface, the exposed skin. Under the surface exists a barrier called the *stratum corneum*, or the horny layer. The *stratum corneum* has been likened to a layer of bricks and mortar, and it is comprised of fats and water. (Remember the fatty acids, with one end of their carbon chain loving water and the other end loathing it? This is a characteristic of the *stratum corneum*.) Any compound that is successful in penetrating the skin's first line of defense usually has the ability to dissolve in both fat and water. If a compound can tiptoe its way through the fats and waters of this external defense membrane, if it can penetrate our outer organ of protection, then it simply passes directly into the bloodstream. In contrast, when we ingest an herb or drug, our liver has a strong say in what our bodies get to experience. Ingested material must have a first pass through the liver, and the liver metabolizes and detoxifies compounds before they enter the bloodstream. Since much of the potency of an herb or drug can be neutralized or diluted by the liver, if a compound gets through the liver at all it is often delivered to the bloodstream in a less concentrated form.

To achieve a therapeutic dosage, it is thus often necessary to ingest a large amount of the herbal or drug constituent, and with larger dosages there is the increased possibility of toxicity. Therefore, if it is possible to deliver a pharmaceutical through the *skin*, a patient can generally achieve a pharmaceutical effect at a lower dosage, the digestive system can be spared the encounter with the drug, and there is a lessened opportunity for toxicity. Again, what is true for drugs is true for herbs.

For a transdermal COX-2 therapy to be useful, it must be easily available and it must work. It must offer the healing powers of the herbs, and provide relief from inflammation.

While it might be wonderfully healing to swim in the calcium- and zinc-rich waters of the Dead Sea, absorbing these minerals in that manner is not practical for most of us. Nor is it practical to swim the Ganges in order to absorb its unusual mica content, or float in the volcanic hot springs of the Arenal volcano in Costa Rica to absorb its mineral wonders. On that last point, the authors have a small organic farm near that volcano, and its waters sound wonderful from our wintry perch in Vermont. But that's for another day . . . .

The key issue is whether the herbal constituents we identified throughout this book will penetrate the skin. The good news is yes, we already have confirmation for

214

some of the featured herbs—ginger, first and foremost. As the opening quotation revealed, ginger extracts have potent transdermal effect, as demonstrated on an arachidonic acid pathway in the Case Western Reserve article. In this study a ginger extract was found to inhibit skin tumors, and research at other international laboratories also confirms the transdermal efficacy of ginger. For example, research from Seoul National University published in *Cancer Letters* in 1998 explained that one of ginger's isolated compounds [*Why can't people just test all 477-plus compounds and see its real magic!?*] a substance called [6]-gingerol, when applied topically "exerts chemoprotective effects through suppression of tumor promotion."

What was particularly interesting about this study was that the researchers compared the topical anti-tumor efficacy of one ginger compound, [6]-gingerol, against another ginger constituent, curcumin. A fragment of ginger was being contrasted to another fragment of ginger! The researchers found that the latter constituent had even greater topical anti-tumor effect than [6]-gingerol. Of course, they failed to compare the isolated compounds against both isolates working together, or against all 477 together. Nonetheless, we do grudgingly acknowledge that the identification of isolated curcumin does have a value. It tells us that turmeric, a cousin to ginger that also contains a high concentration of curcumin, has the ability to topically inhibit cancer. This is consistent with research from 1987 that an ointment of curcumin from turmeric was "found to produce remarkable symptomatic relief in patients with external cancerous lesions." More recently, 1998 research from the National Institute of Nutrition in India reported that a "paint" or topical application of turmeric "may have a plausible chemopreventative effect on oral pre-cancerous lesions."

Turning our attention back to ancient Greece, in our consideration of Hippocrates' prescription of white willow bark for fever and inflammation you may recall that we noted that the bark of the white willow, *Salix alba*, contains salicylates that inhibit COX-2. As a German medical publication reported in 1993, both salicylates and salicylic acid can be used topically and can penetrate into deeper tissue layers.

Green tea contains salicylic acid, so we have another confirmed topical COX-2 inhibitor; and the State University of New York and Rutgers University reported in 1994 that topical application of rosemary constituents—ursolic acid and carnosol—inhibited mouse skin tumors by forty-five to sixty-one percent. Remember that holy basil also contains ursolic acid? Add two more to the topical COX-2 list.

We promise to keep reviewing the medical research to find verification of the topical COX-2 and anti-tumor effects of the other herbs we have highlighted. Our

216

continuing research on this and herbal COX-2 inhibition in general will be posted at www.cox-2reduction.com, and we invite scientists open to the healing powers of herbs to add their research to the site so that it becomes a clearinghouse of the most recent information in this field. We also hope that this analysis of transdermal herbalism stimulates researchers to confirm in their laboratories the topical values of these time-tested herbs. Moreover, we are absolutely confident that the proven topical inhibition of COX-2 and the inhibition of tumors by ginger, turmeric, green tea, holy basil and rosemary is not anomalous. There is simply no reason to believe, for example, that *Scutellaria*, which can rapidly enter and rescue dying heart tissue and cross the blood/brain barrier, cannot penetrate the skin. Western science is already stirring, already waking up to the COX-2 inhibiting effects of these herbs, and it is just a matter of time before their transdermal effects are confirmed.

NOW, FOR A FINAL LEAP

One of the great joys of studying herbs is the inherently international flavor of the quest. Mother Nature has placed healing herbs all around the world, as if to ensure that people from every culture and region will have access to Her intelligence. When master herbalists from other cultures come to North America, they want to study the traditional medical systems of

Native Americans. Such openness to other cultures led to the discovery, for example, of the use of saw palmetto, *Serenoa repens*, as an aphrodisiac by Native Americans in southeast U.S., which stimulated the research on saw palmetto for prostate health. Openness, an unbounded approach, a willingness to explore other cultures and other systems, these are the hallmarks of master herbalists discovering new expressions of nature's wisdom.

In the next part of this chapter we invite you to become an apprentice master herbalist, and leave the boundaries of your ordinary thinking behind. We invite you to take a journey into the realm of herbalism through the sense of smell, which we now call aromatherapy.

Again, we are not introducing a new concept. In Ayurveda, doctors called *vaidyas* have burned herbs to release their healing powers into the wind. The burning of incense has traditionally been used for healing and purification, as well as for sacramental purposes. In Hindu ceremonies, the offering of *dhupam*, of incense, is said to purify the air. In Jewish and Catholic ceremonies, worshipers are invited to smell special spices, some burning, in ornamental spice boxes or incense holders. Does this have only sacramental purpose? Consider that frankincense, also known as Boswellia, contains a compound called boswellic acid that is known to inhibit COX-2 inflammatory processes. In fact, there are Ayurvedic joint and arthritic preparations that feature

218

Boswellia. Perhaps the three wise men, who were Zoroastrian priests from Persia, had this in mind when giving the gift of frankincense.

As we mentioned earlier in this book, rosemary has been burned for thousands of years in Greece to stimulate the mind. Students would also put sprigs in their hair to improve their concentration. Rosemary was often burnt in churches of the Middle Ages, hence its other name, *incensier*. Rosemary is one of the great COX-2 herbal inhibitors, and its consistent, historic use aromatically strongly supports the anti-inflammatory value of its aroma.

Then there is the fragrance industry; the frenzy to find pheromones (forgive the alliteration!); the use of fragrances to attract or repel animals. We know that fragrances have a powerful effect. The essential oils stimulate the sensitive nerve receptors in the nose and sinuses, and the "message" of the herb goes directly into our consciousness. Here's a test to prove that, which one of the authors has used on himself countless times. Take a rose with sweet fragrance and inhale deeply. At the same time, try to think an ugly thought. Can't be done! The mind becomes so saturated with the bliss of the rose's essential oil that the consciousness changes. Such a fragrance only supports joyous thoughts. At least it has that effect on us.

Other less pleasant aromas can cause the body to

tense, the pulse to race, the blood pressure to rise, and cause an increased production of stress hormones. Animals can smell predators, and the smell alone can stimulate a fight or flight reaction. Animals can also smell fear, and know that they are not in danger.

It is too late in the day for anyone to deny the relationship between mind and body. We all recognize that anxiety and depression create illness, and as for happiness, the famous English writer and clergyman Robert Burton observed almost four hundred years ago that "humor purges the blood, making the body young and lively, and fit for any manner of employment." Today, that observation has become a science—the new science of psychoneuroimmunology, which studies how emotions affect the immune system. This is not just a "Comedy Club" quote masquerading as science, but a serious study by highly educated scholars of what we think is totally obvious: People who are happy are healthier, have stronger immune systems, and have less pain.

And certain fragrances, through history, have stimulated specific mental states that promote proper mental and physical functioning, such as the traditional burning of rosemary to promote heightened mental clarity and memory. So much for the general introduction to the concept of aromatherapy.

Now, for the fun part. The authors acknowledge up

front that we are not trained clinical aromatherapists, but we have employed its healing and soothing principles in our own lives to great effect. In undertaking to make recommendations for aromas to reduce inflammation, we thus sought the advice of experts in the field, and we were fortunate to have obtained the counsel of Jane Buckle, one of the world's premier aromatherapists. Working with us, she has suggested four essential oils that have, in her clinical experience and studies, reduced inflammation and brought relief to people suffering from arthritis and other conditions of chronic pain.

FOUR ESSENTIAL OILS –
JANE BUCKLE'S RECOMMENDATIONS

Black Pepper. This was a bit of a surprise to us as well, but Jane explained that persons with fibromyalgia have responded well to this essential oil when it is part of a mixture. Black pepper, or *Piper nigrum*, is native to India but is now cultivated in many tropical countries. This plant is a woody vine with heart-shaped leaves and small white flowers. It begins to create berries after three to four years, and the berries gradually turn from red to black.

Black pepper has long been prized for its healing properties. Atilla the Hun demanded three thousand pounds of pepper in ransom for Rome, and Theophrastus and Hippocrates refer to its medicinal uses. Pliny observed that pepper was more expensive than gold. It has had many traditional medical uses, one interesting one being its use for gonorrhea. Jane mentioned to us that "the idea of using black pepper for venereal diseases does bring tears to my eyes!"

The color of essential oil of black pepper is clear to pale olive. Chemically, it is up to 90% sesquiterpenes. Its aromatherapeutic applications include use for muscle fatigue, arthritis, neuralgia, fibromyalgia, and as an analgesic (for pain relief).

Spike Lavender. Spike lavender, *Lavandula latifolia,* is suggested by the British Herbal Pharmacopoeia for rheumatic pain. Its essential oil has been used on paralyzed limbs, stiff joints and sprains.

It grows wild in Spain and France, but is cultivated worldwide. An evergreen shrub with broad leaves and dull grayish flowers, it is taller than true lavender. Its essential oil is colorless to pale yellow, and contains cineole and camphor among its chemical constituents.

Lemongrass. This herb grows in tropical climates, and the particular variety recommended is *Cymbopogon citratus,* which is also known as West Indian lemongrass. The herb and its essential oils have been used in East Indian culture for hundreds of years. Lemongrass tea is used as a febrifuge, or a temperature reducer, which is consistent with its anti-inflammatory effects. The aroma is gently lemony, and mixes well with the aromas of spike lavender, black pepper and rosemary (the final recommended essential oil.) Jane has determined that lemongrass essential oil is useful for muscular pain, and its recognized uses are, among others, as an analgesic, an antipyretic and a relaxant.

Rosemary. We seem to always return to rosemary, the dew of the sea. Jane reports that she has had great success with using rosemary essential oil in post-viral fatigue syndrome (patients ache all over), as well as for sports injuries and arthritic pain.

Rosemary is a favorite of the fragrance industry. Hungary Water, made from rosemary, is widely used in making perfumes.

Its aromatherapy applications include use as an anti-inflammatory, for memory loss, alertness, as an anti-depressant, and for enhancing neuromuscular tone.

ESSENTIAL OIL EXTRACTION ISSUES

By this point you can predict that we would not recommend the use of any chemical solvents, ever. Accordingly, these essential oils should be extracted by steam distillation or supercritical extraction.

HOW TO DERIVE THE BENEFITS
OF ESSENTIAL OILS

The manner of mixing, blending and utilization of any essential oils will be a personal decision. Both authors have small waterfalls in our offices, and from time to time we drop the essential oils into the water and enjoy the fragrances as they diffuse into the atmosphere. There are many types of fragrance diffusers available on the market today.

Pure essential oils can, if mixed in just the right proportion with the proper cream base, be used topically. We do not, however, recommend that you do this at home unless you have serious familiarity and competency with the topical use of essential oils. They are wonderful friends, but they sometimes have an "attitude" if not handled with care. On the other hand, if handled properly and put in the right cream and herbal base, the fragrances create a wonderful effect that augments the anti-inflammatory properties of the herbal COX-2 inhibitors as applied topically. We have mixed up such a topical ointment, and it is a blessing!

As another word of caution, we would be remiss not to strongly remind you that since pure essential oils are highly concentrated we only recommend them for internal consumption under the guidance of a trained health professional.

UNBOUNDED HEALING

For some of you, the idea of stimulating healing through the subtle mechanism of aroma may be a bit of a stretch. Your habits of thought may tell you that smelling flowers and essential oils is too subtle, too insubstantial, to have any real effect. But to be perfectly blunt, those habits of thought may have led you to inflammation, imbalance and illness. It's time to try new thoughts, or maybe just stop thinking and start enjoying the softer impulses of life. For life is an adventure, and boundaries, especially boundaries of thought, are boring.

We firmly believe that the essential oils of herbs, flowers and spices can uplift the spirit, mind and body, and we urge you to follow the advice of King Solomon when he spoke to his beloved in the *Song of Songs*:

> Until the day breaths
> and the shadows flee,
> I will hie me to the mountain of myrrh
> and the hill of frankincense.

And if, before your daylight comes, you still won't go to those hills and mountains of fragrance, listen to Alice when she went through the looking glass into a garden of live flowers:

> This time she came upon a large flower-bed,
> with a border of daisies,
> and a willow-tree growing in the middle.

225

"Oh, Tiger-lily!" said Alice, addressing herself
to one that was waving gracefully about in the wind,
"I *wish* you could talk!"
"We can talk," said the Tiger-lily,
"when there's anybody worth talking to."

CHAPTER TWENTY-THREE

Final Considerations:
Physical & Metaphysical

Samson, as he prays for death:
O! that torment should not be confin'd
To the body's wounds and sores,
With maladies innumerable
In heart, head, breast, and reins;
But must secret passage find
To th' inmost mind,
There exercise all his fierce accidents,
And on her purest spirits prey
As on entrails, joints, and limbs;
With answerable pain, but more intense,
Though void of corporal sense.
My griefs not only pain me
As a lingering disease,
But finding no redress, ferment and rage,
Nor less than wounds immedicable
Rankle, and fester, and gangrene,
To black mortification.
Thoughts my tormentors, arm'd with deadly stings,
Mangle my apprehensive tenderest parts;
Exasperate, exulcerate, and raise
Dire inflammation which no cooling herb
Or med'cinal liquor can assuage.

—*Samson Agonistes*, John Milton

Samson, blinded and chained, tortured and taunted, yet his real grief is the torment of thought. His own thoughts sting and mangle him, and raise an inflammation "which no cooling herb or med'cinal liquor can assuage."

We agree. Some malaise is too deep to be "cured" by herbs alone. We love these precious plants, and have spent the greater part of our collective lives growing and studying them. As we mentioned, we have an organic farm in Costa Rica, we make herbal extracts in our homes, and our lives are devoted to the powerful healing science of traditional medicine. Even so, herbs cannot be expected, on their own, to soothe every pain in our flesh, bones and souls. We each must shoulder some of that responsibility, and thus work in concert with the herbs that nature has kindly offered to us.

The option to take the strongest pharmaceutical drug agents we can find and go for the sure-fire quick fix, the chemical "certainty," always remains open. Anyone can simply opt to blast the pain, to anesthetize the body and not deal with the deeper issues. That's one strategy for life, and sometimes, when things are truly dire, it seems like the only choice. We are reminded, though, of one of our favorite lines in modern literature from the Tom Stoppard play, *Rosenkrantz and Guildenstern are Dead*. Here a destitute and pathetic stage actor explains that "all the money we had we lost betting on certainties." Taking synthetic chemicals on a chronic basis to ease pain and inflammation can be a losing "bet on a certainty," which is certainly not a wager that we would choose to lightly make. We would rather bet on nature, and ourselves.

In contrast to the quick-fix approach, you now have the knowledge of the herbs that can, on a deep enzymatic level, help heal the broken physiology. Your first step, then, should be to act on that knowledge and obtain these herbs for your personal use. Keep in mind, however, that Samson is right. It is not enough to have *only* these cooling herbs. What else we recommend, by way of healing the torment of thought, will be touched upon shortly later. For now, however, let's start with the herbs and highlight some guideposts to be aware of as you enter this fascinating world of herbal medicine.

BROAD SPECTRUM

We advocate using broad-spectrum herbal extracts. We believe that a reliable extract can assure you that the constituents you are looking for in an herb are present, and are in a potency that gives you confidence in the herb's effect.

NOT "STANDARDIZED"

We do not suggest that you look for standardized herbs that isolate and concentrate one phytochemical ingredient. Ginger has 477 constituents, not just [6]-gingerol, for example. Turmeric has hundreds of ingredients, not just curcumin. Green tea has hundreds of ingredients, not just epigallocatechin-gallate. If you buy an extract that is "standardized" to one particular isolated ingredient, you are buying something more like a drug than a complex herb. It is the difference between listening to one person screaming one word versus listening to a chorus gently singing. Go for the chorus.

USE THE HERBS TOGETHER

To maximize the herbal benefits, use herbs "singing" together. Early on in this book we compared the pharmaceutical COX-2 inhibitors to a silver bullet, and recommended a more comprehensive strategy. As we've pointed out before, Celebrex and Vioxx are each simply one synthetic molecule that inhibits the COX-2 enzyme in one particular way. They are unquestionably very powerful silver bullets, and represent a form of human engineering genius that we respect. But, we must recognize that such engineering genius is limited.

In contrast, in using herbs we approach COX-2 inhibition from multiple complex directions; and these herbs embody a vastly more impressive intelligence—the very wisdom of nature. It is to our advantage to use these bundles of nature's intelligence in concert, so that their capabilities work synergistically. On that point, you may recall that the research demonstrates that green tea and turmeric are powerful COX-2 inhibitors in their own right, but if taken together they magnify each other's effects. We want to maximize those synergistic opportunities.

THE HERBS SHOULD ALSO
BE USED ON THEIR OWN

After all, each of the herbs discussed in this book has myriad constituents and represents, in the microcosm of that one plant, the type of synergy that we seek. Ginger has multiple constituents including curcumin, melatonin, kaempferol. Rosemary has apigenin and ursolic acid. Holy basil has ursolic acid and cortisol-reducing compounds. Green tea has multiple catechins, phenols, and so on. They are their own bundles of synergistic ingredients, so we should feel comfortable using them on their own. Green tea: drink it often, preferably daily. Ginger: cook with it, drink teas and tonics made from it, take a bath with it, and take it as a supplement. Holy basil: where there's stress, there should be holy basil. We need as much balance in life as possible, and holy basil helps. Rosemary: one of our favorite uses is still the topical application on the head.

Embrace each individual herb, but also take them together.

JUST SAY NO TO CHEMICAL SOLVENTS!

Hexane may be useful in removing oils and spots from clothing, but there are other ways to extract the phytonutrients from herbs. The same is true for acetone and other potentially toxic chemical solvents. When these type of solvents are used in extraction, one of two things usually happens: (1) some of the solvent remains in the extract, and you end up ingesting a dangerous chemical; or (2) the extract is heated to facilitate the removal of the chemical solvent, which puts a temperature stress on the herb and may alter its properties. In short, we are exposed to enough synthetic chemicals in our environment; we don't need to use them or potentially ingest them on the herbs we take.

DON'T USE HERBS
THAT ARE ENDANGERED SPECIES

Some herbs have been over-harvested and are now endangered. Buy from companies that are committed to sustainable agriculture and to protecting endangered herbal species. In time, these endangered herbs may recover sufficiently to allow us to take them in good conscience. None of the herbs we have featured in this book are endangered.

LOOK FOR EXTRACTS MADE
SUPERCRITICALLY

Supercritical extraction is a relatively new method. It is useful for herbs that are oily in nature, like ginger, rosemary, oregano, kava, St. John's Wort, saw palmetto, feverfew, and the like. The process uses compressed carbon dioxide gas, which is an excellent dissolver of the oily fractions of the herbs. The process does not involve heating the herbs to high temperatures, and when the pressure is released the carbon dioxide just goes back into the atmosphere. No environmental pollution, no chemicals, no temperature stress on the herb, and best of all the process can extract an extremely broad spectrum of the oily, resinous constituents. (To obtain a good representation of plant constituents that are not dissolved by pressurized CO_2, other non-solvent extraction techniques can be used.)

To give you an idea of the concentrated power of the supercritical extraction process, it takes 250 pounds of fresh ginger to yield 1 pound of the supercritical extract. The extract is thus not only free of any solvents, it is extraordinarily concentrated and broad spectrum. Moreover, certain CO_2 extracts and constituents demonstrate unusual shelf stability, such as the resinous hyperforins (the highly active plant constituents) of a supercritical St. John's Wort extract. The hyperforin resins are generally quite unstable when alcohol-extracted, which is unfortunate as they are a broad fraction of St. John's Wort constituents that dramatically help treat depression. Fortunately, the supercritical process yields a highly-concentrated, broad-spectrum, and extremely stable representation of hyperforins.

233

BE GUIDED BY RESPECTED EXPERTS

These COX-2 inhibiting herbs, individually and in formulas, are already available from healthcare practitioners and natural food and vitamin stores. We believe that this book, the continuing educational efforts by such champion herbalists as Dr. James Duke, and the general awareness of the critical importance of COX-2 inhibition will no doubt stimulate even more herbal products designed to safely reduce inappropriate COX-2 inflammation and its disease expressions: arthritis, cancer and Alzheimer's disease. To find the proper products for you, we always suggest obtaining guidance from a knowledgeable herbal expert. Who those people are will vary from community to community and nation to nation, so there is no one "seal of approval" we can offer. But, if you do your homework you may find the knowledgeable healer you are looking for in your own physician's office, with your chiropractor, naturopath, Ayurvedic specialist, physical therapist, or with other complementary healthcare practitioners. You may wish to consult with the American Herbalists Guild, American Botanical Council, Herb Research Foundation or any of the other resources listed in the appendix at the end of the book. You may also find a fountain of herbal expertise in your neighborhood natural food/vitamin store, where some of the owners or staff have trained and studied for years to be able to guide you. Today, you may also find the required expertise, products and guidance on the Internet. The information is there, and dedicated herbal experts can be found. Ask them for herbal formulations for COX-2 inhibition, and be guided by their knowledge. This book represents information on herbal COX-2 reduction that is current through the date of its publication. In order to be able to continue to provide you with current information on the extraordinary health benefits being discovered every day with respect to herbal COX-2 reduction, we have created a website, noted earlier, to serve as a clearinghouse of this information. This website, www.cox2reduction.com, will gather and present the newest stories and scientific abstracts on the developing revolution of herbal COX-2 reduction. We look forward to seeing you there.

A FINAL LESSON IN UNBOUNDED HEALING

In the last chapter, we urged you to be open to the subtle healing forces in essential plant oils. Many surgeons and hospitals are beginning to utilize these essential oils to facilitate recovery and healing. In so doing they have taken a step away from the strictures of "conventional" thinking, and taken a step toward unbounded patient care. You need to take that step as well—for yourself and for your family.

In addition to the herbs, essential oils and fatty acids that we have recommended for COX-2 inhibition, we can introduce several other healing forces into our lives to tame the beast of inflammation and restore health and balance.

- **First, we need to drink water.** Pure water, and more of it than you think. Most have heard that we need eight glasses a day—that is a good beginning. We think you should drink one tall glass of fresh, pure water every hour. It replenishes the body and cleanses the system.

- **Second, engage in regular exercise.** It doesn't have to be strenuous, but if that brings you pleasure then so be it. You will know the level of activity that is right when you reach it, but you need to move. Your form of exercise can be hiking or walking, but it must get your blood flowing, your muscles pumping, and your lungs working. Again, it doesn't mean you *have* to huff and puff; you just have to move.

- **Third, eat wholesome, nourishing, fresh food, especially fruits and vegetables.** If possible, these foods should be organically grown. Scientists are also becoming aware that certain conditions of inflammation can be aggravated by eating foods that are incompatible with your body and lifestyle. For additional information on how to eat in accordance with your

236

unique characteristics and requirements, we list some resources in the appendix.

- **Fourth, laugh.** Patch Adams was right. Laughter is one of the best healing forces on earth. If mental boundaries are boring, then brooding in chronic sadness is an insult to life. Life is to enjoy, and joy is a wonderful healing force.

- **Fifth, sunlight is not a bad thing.** Sunshine is wonderful for you in moderation, just don't oxidize your flesh and create reactive oxygen species. But fresh air and sunshine heal. They prevent disease. So go outside and breathe.

- **Sixth, be a gardener.** Gardening connects you to the earth. In a wonderful book by Walker Percy called *Love in the Ruins,* a doctor came up with a treatment for a man who felt powerless, alienated and consumed in thought. The prescription? Roll up your pants, take off your shoes and socks, and walk in the Louisiana swamps every day. Get totally grounded and simple.

This program worked wonders for the patient. We have always found that getting our hands in cool, sweet soil is great medicine.

- **Seventh, seek knowledge.** This book does not

attempt to be the comprehensive guide for all the programs and strategies available for handling the disease expressions of inappropriate COX-2 inflammation. Other extensive reference works are now available. We believe that knowledge is a powerful healing force in its own right. You may find these reference works in your libraries, at bookstores and health food stores, and on the Internet. We provide a list of useful reference works in an appendix at the back of this book.

- **Eighth, love**. Samson felt alienated from man, from the world, from God. Love unites, and extinguishes separation. So, make love to your beloved, hug your children, call your parents, and care about the world.

- **Ninth, use support.** You obviously lean on your family and those dear to you, but you also have experienced and caring healthcare practitioners to help guide you toward health. They come by many names—chiropractors, medical doctors (both conventional and complementary), naturopaths, massage therapists, acupuncturists, herbalists, and others.

- **Ten, make silence your medicine.** We have just recommended walking, hugging, laughing, gardening and breathing. We also recommend silence. The deepest inflammation in Samson's life was his separation from that supreme peace that lies within. Instead, the noise of his thoughts and doubts enchained him. We can relate to that type of imprisonment. Maybe this is the reason for the enduring fascination with Samson. When we were young we thought ourselves invincible. Success was to be ours, and we were certain to find the way. But, somewhere along the way we stumbled. We could not clearly see the path, and we became chained to our conditions. Then our self-doubts and despair consumed us, gradually taking their toll on our bodies. Inflammation, everywhere. Could this be the metaphor, the true enduring lesson, of Samson's life?

Maybe we try to read too much into Milton's masterpiece, but we believe that a reality of life today is the reality of Samson. A reality of inflammation so profound that it consumes the body and mind in fire. Rampant cancer, epidemic arthritis, and millions slowly succumbing to inflammation that steals the mind—this is a sad truth of modern life. We believe with all our hearts that there is a more sublime value in life that will, on the deepest levels, extinguish the inflammation.

Are we suggesting a spiritual journey? Of course. What other journey is there, after all? Your humble authors became friends almost thirty years ago. Now our wives and children are friends as well. And we have been meditating for almost thirty years, although we are surely novices in that regard. But we are on the path. If, as the Irish poet Yeats once wrote, our minds are torn by the "ravens of unresting thought," there is also the mystical promise of attaining a state of quiet peace where the mind is "like a lamp that does not flicker in a windless place."

May you all find that peace, for in that quietness true healing can occur.

APPENDIX A

Historical and Current Ethnobotanical Uses of COX-2 Inhibiting Herbs

This book has focused almost exclusively on the COX-2 inhibiting properties of the featured herbs. We could have written a complete book on each of the herbs covered here, describing their other medicinal properties and usages, but that was not our task. It is worthwhile to remember, however, that due to the biochemical complexity of these herbs, we obtain not only their COX-2 inhibiting benefits but many other life-supporting features. What follows is a brief look, really only a glimpse, at the other traditional medicinal uses of the COX-2 inhibiting herbs.

Barberry—*Berberis vulgaris*

Barberry has been used throughout the ages for a multitude of inflammatory disorders including arthritis, and various types of tumors (most notably, liver, neck and stomach). In Mongolia it was used to treat mucus disorders; in Iran it was employed as a breath freshener and tonic. The American Indians had a wealth of uses for barberry, including blood purification, coughs, consumption, weakness, heartburn, lack of appetite, kidney disorders, rheumatism, sores and ulcers. Russians have used it to treat inflammation, hemorrhage, gallbladder disorders and hypertension, to increase bile production, and to regulate female hormones.

Duke, J.A., Ph.D. *CRC Handbook of Medicinal Herbs*. Boca Raton, Florida: CRC Press, 1985.

Chinese Goldthread—*Coptis chinensis*

This herb has been utilized for two thousand years in China to treat many conditions, including internal and external inflammations, such as inflammation of the mouth and tongue, and inflammatory bowel disease. Other applications of Chinese goldthread include the treatment of burns, rashes, eye and ear irritations (such as conjunctivitis and otitis media), yeast infections, dysentery, diarrhea, acute enteritis, coughs, tuberculosis, typhoid, diphtheria, scarlet fever, delirium due to high fever, high blood pressure, high cholesterol, low bile

242

production and leukemia. It is also considered helpful in cases of mental restlessness and irritation, insomnia and fidgeting.

"Coptis rhizome." <http://www.techno-shaman.com/store/ingredients/coptis.htm>

Yeung, H., C.A., O.M.D., Ph.D. *Handbook of Chinese Herbs and Formulas, Vol. 1.* Los Angeles: Institute of Chinese Medicine, 1985.

Feverfew—*Tanacetum parthenium*

Feverfew, which is native to the Balkan Peninsula, has been used in Greece since the first century for relief from headache, stomach ailments, fevers and menstrual irregularities. These seem to be common uses for feverfew, as the people of Central and South America, Costa Rica and Mexico similarly used it for many of those same conditions. Additionally, it was used in Central and South America to ease morning sickness and to treat kidney pains. In the United Kingdom, feverfew is used to treat vertigo and joint inflammation associated with rheumatism and arthritis. In Venezuela it is recommended for earaches.

Foster, S. *Feverfew; Tanacetum parthenium.* Austin, Texas: American Botanical Council, 1996.

Foster, S. "Feverfew: When the Head Hurts." *Alternative & Complementary Therapies,* Sept./Oct. 1995, pp. 335-337.

Ginger—*Zingiber officinale*

Ginger has been, and is currently, used for a vast

assortment of ailments. Ginger was used to promote wound healing and counter the pain and heat (fever) of inflammatory disorders in many countries including Brazil, China, India, Indonesia, New Guinea, Sudan and Thailand. One of ginger's most common uses is as a digestive tonic. It is employed for that purpose by many cultures, including Mexico, Papua-New Guinea, India and Fiji. Ginger has also been acknowledged as an emmenagogue, contraceptive and aphrodisiac by the people of China, Cuba and India. Ginger is considered beneficial for morning sickness, childbirth, and as a post-birth tonic by the people of England, Sumatra and Malaysia, respectively. Some of its more unusual uses include treatment for snakebite (Indonesia) and poisonous stings (Papua-New Guinea), and for promotion of hair growth (Japan).

Schulick, P. *Ginger: Common Spice & Wonder Drug*. Brattleboro, Vermont: Herbal Free Press, 1994.

Gotu Kola—*Centella asiatica*

As an illustration of the widespread use of *gotu kola*, consider the many locations where it was employed as a therapeutic herb: India, Pakistan, Malaysia, parts of Eastern Europe, China, Indonesia, Australia, Sri Lanka, the South Pacific, Madagascar, and the southern half of Africa. *Gotu kola* is revered as an herb for longevity by the people of Sri Lanka—they noted the fact that elephants, known for their long life span, eat this plant regularly. It is believed that a Chinese herbalist, namely Li Ching Yun, supposedly lived 256 years due to his frequent use of this plant! It is not surprising then, that China also praises this herb for enhancing longevity, in addition to their use of it for many other conditions, such as depression, fevers, leukorrhea, boils, fractions, contusions and strains. India has many applications for *gotu kola* as well, including its use in cases of leprosy, lupus and psoriasis, and for general wound healing. It is considered a brain and nerve tonic in India as well, and they use it to improve the quality of spiritual meditations.

Anonymous. "Centella asiatica (Gotu kola)." *American Journal of Natural Medicine,* July/August 1996, Vol. 3, No. 6, pp. 22-25.

"Gotu Kola Fact Sheet."<http://www.americahealth.com/Gotu.html>

"Gotu Kola - Facts and Information." <http://www.go-symmetry.com/gotu-kola.htm>

"Gotu Kola: The Spiritual Herb - Herb Notes Volume 10." <http://www.frontierherb.com/herbs/notes/herbs.notes.no10.html>

"Gotu Kola." <http://www.theherbalist.com/gotakola.htm>

"Herbal Information Center - Gotu Kola - Herbs." <http://www.kcweb.com/herb/gotu.htm>

"Medicinal Plants." <http://www.niam.com/centella.htm>

Green Tea—*Camellia sinensis*

According to one legend, green tea was discovered by a Chinese emperor in 2700 B.C.E. As he sat in the forest next to a wild tea plant drinking a cup of hot water, a leaf from the tea plant happened to drop in his cup and he immediately savored the taste. Historically, green tea has been used in China as treatment for multiple health complaints—including headaches, body cramps, fatigue and depression. Japanese use of green tea has a rich history as well. From 800 C.E. on, Buddhist monks in Japan used green tea to stay awake during meditation. The Japanese tea ceremony associates the drinking of green tea with spiritual harmony and rejuvenation. In India, green tea is used as an astringent, stimulant and diuretic.

"Green Tea (Camellia sinensis)." <http://www.mothernature.com/ency/Herb/Green_Tea.asp>

Knight, J. "Reading the Tea Leaves." *Herbs for Health* May/June 1998: 41-45.

McCaleb, R. "Teas for Good Health." *Delicious!* Oct.1996.

Snow, J. Herbal Monograph: *"Camellia sinensis* (L.) Kuntze (Theaceae)." *The Protocol Journal of Botanical Medicine* Autumn 1995, pp. 47-51.

Holy Basil—*Ocimum sanctum*

In its native country, India, this plant is called *tulsi* or *tulasi* (which means "matchless"), and it is found everywhere in ancient Hindu literature. Following the endorsement of one of their holiest figures, Lord Vishnu, many believed holy basil was truly holy—some devoted their lives to growing, protecting and maintaining this single botanical. Beads were made out of the basil plant and worn as necklaces in order to increase religious faith and longevity. Holy basil was used for systemic support, and for treatment of numerous conditions, including asthma, bronchitis, the fevers of cholera, influenza, malaria, and to treat cancer. Other cultures have found uses for holy basil, including treatment of arthritis and inflammation (Egypt) and for nerves and fainting spells (Rome).

"Ayurvedic Herb: Tulasi (*Ocimum sanctum*)." *Ayurveda Monthly Newletter.* Colorado Springs, Colo.: Living Wholeness, 1997.

The Indian Materia Medica.

Majeed, M., Ph.D. and L. Prakash, Ph.D. *Ocimum Sanctum.* Piscataway, New Jersey: Sabinsa Corporation, 1998.

Hops—*Humulus lupulus*

Hops are native to England, and have also been extensively cultivated in Germany, South America, France, Australia and the United States. The Latin name is of uncertain origin, but it is thought that *humulus* was derived from *humus*, reflecting the moist, rich ground in which the plant grows. The name *lupulus* is a bit more sinister, as it comes from the Latin for "wolf." The plant is a powerful climbing, twining herb, and it was thought to strangle its neighbors like a wolf. The name "hops" comes from the Anglo-Saxon *hoppan*, which means "climbing," again referring to the plant's growth pattern. The Spanish name for hops is *flores de cerveza*, literally "flowers of beer."

Although perhaps most widely recognized as a primary ingredient in brewing and flavoring beer, the medicinal properties of hops have been valued for centuries. The Romans used hops as a nerve tonic and sedative. The sedative effects of hops were recognized when hops pickers seemed to tire easily (due to the transference of hop resin, most likely the humulone content, from their hands to their mouths and via transdermal delivery directly to the bloodstream). Pillows filled with warm hops have been traditionally used to encourage sleep, and were valued for providing relief from toothaches and earaches. Poultices of hops are used topically to treat sores, muscle spasms and to reduce local inflammation. Hops is considered soothing to the stomach—it has been used to control diarrhea and irritable bowel syndrome. In Sweden, a durable cloth is made from the fibers of hops, and paper can be made from the stem.

Lust, J. *The Herb Book.* New York: Bantam Books, 1974.

Grieve, M. *A Modern Herbal, Vol. 1.* New York: Dover Publications, 1971.

Wilen, J. and L. Wilen *Live and Be Well.* New York: HarperCollins, 1992,

Hops – MotherNature.com Health Encyclopedia www.mothernature.com

Hops – Herbal Materia Medica/Health World Online www.healthworld.com

Hops. www.botanical.com

Hu zhang—*Polygonum cuspidatum*

Originally from East Asia, other names for this herb include "knotweed" and "tiger cane." In China it has been used for over two thousand years for such ailments as arthritic pain, respiratory inflammations, and to promote wound healing. In Japan, *hu zhang* has been used for skin irritations and to counteract multiple infectious agents.

Leung, A.Y. and S. Foster. "Skullcap, Baikal (Huangqin)." *Encyclopedia of Common Natural Ingredients.* 2nd ed., 1996, pp. 554-555.

Oregano—*Origanum vulgare*

Native to the Mediterranean, this herb was first used by the ancient Greeks, who named it *origanos* meaning, "delight or joy of the mountains." Its use spread throughout Europe as a treatment for respiratory inflammation—and is also used as a sedative and diuretic. In China, oregano is used for fevers, digestive irritation and skin inflammation. Use of this herb gained popularity in the United States around 1930 to treat indigestion and nausea. It also appears in that literature as an herb of choice effective for respiratory and skin irritations and to treat arthritis, ear pain or ringing, toothache and nervousness.

Kloss, J. *Back to Eden.* Santa Barbara, Calif.: Woodbridge Press, 1939.

Leung, A. Y. and S. Foster. "Oregano." *Encyclopedia of Common Natural Ingredients.* 2nd Ed., 1996, pp. 398-399.

"Oil of Oregano Product Review." <http://www.droregano.net/ooregano.html>

Rosemary—*Rosmarinus officinalis*

Originally from the Mediterranean region, the name rosemary comes from *ros marininus*, or the "dew of the sea." It was widely used throughout history for its mentally stimulating properties and its ability to preserve meats. Rosemary was one of the main ingredients of "Hungary water," a lauded lotion favorite to Queen Elizabeth of Hungary. Supposedly, the queen first received the liquor from a monk when, at the age of seventy-two, she was gouty and paralytic. After applying it every day, she fully recovered her health and beauty. This apparently helped her to win the King of Poland as a husband. The use of rosemary for health purposes is widespread. In Brazil, it is used to treat respiratory irritations like asthma and bronchitis; in Cuba for fever, hoarseness and insomnia; in Latin America for digestive complaints, edema and arthritic complaints. Interestingly, rosemary is most widely recognized as a memory aid— it has been used for that purpose in the traditions of Greece, England, Rome and the Middle East.

Duke, J.A., Ph.D. *CRC Handbook of Medicinal Herbs*. Boca Raton, Florida: CRC Press, 1985.

Ingram, Dr. C. "Juice of Rosemary." <http://www.droregano.net/jrosemary.html>

Ingram, Dr. C. "Oil of Rosemary." <http://www.droregano.net/orosemary.html>

Jones, C., Ph.D. "Rosemary's Whole-Plant Properties Counter Cancer." *Health & Nutrition Breakthroughs*. July 1998: 34-35.

Lavabre, M. *Aromatherapy Workbook.* Rochester, Vermont: Healing Arts Press, 1990.

"Remember Rosemary." <http://www.suite101.com/article.cfm/herb_gardening/6368>

"Rosemary (Rosmarinus officinalis)." <http://www.mothernature.com/ency/Herb/Rosemary.asp>

Scutellaria—*Scutellaria baicalensis*

Native to eastern Asia, this herb is also termed "baikal skullcap." Since 1065 B.C.E., *Scutellaria* has been used in China for many health conditions—including the treatment of restlessness, throat pains, cough, chest pains and headache. It has also been used to treat facial inflammation, reduce fevers, chills, nausea, vomiting, indigestion and diarrhea. Other Chinese uses of *Scutellaria* include treatment of dysentery, blood and mucous in the stool, skin irritations and the promotion of wound healing, and the correction of cardiac abnormalities.

Hsu, H., Ph.D., and C. Hsu, Ph.D. *Commonly Used Chinese Herb Formulas with Illustrations.* Long Beach, Calif.: Oriental Healing Arts Institute, 1980.

Leung, A.Y. and S. Foster. "Skullcap, Baikal (Huangqin)." *Encyclopedia of Common Natural Ingredients.* 2nd Ed, 1996, pp. 554-555.

Reid, D.P. *Chinese Herbal Medicine.* Boston: Shambhala Publications, 1987.

Turmeric—*Curcuma longa*

Native to India and a cousin to ginger, turmeric is widely used as a food preservative and spice for foods such as curry and mustard. In China (where it is recorded to have been used since the seventh century) and India, turmeric is used to treat a multitude of health conditions including systemic inflammation, blood disorders, chest pain, liver disorders, skin lesions and menstrual difficulties. In India, turmeric salves are applied to the skin of small-pox sufferers.

Blumenthal, M. "From Curry to the Curious Curcuminoids." *Whole Foods* July 1996: 78-82.

Kuttan, R., et al. "Potential Anticancer Activity of Turmeric (*Curcuma longa*)." *Cover Letters* 18 June 1985: 197-202.

Kuttan, R., P.C. Sudheeran and C.D. Josph. "Turmeric and Curcumin as Topical Agents in Cancer Therapy." *Tumori* 5 Nov. 1985: 29-31.

McMahon, S.L. "Turmeric: from Kitchen Cabinet to Medicine Chest." *Vegetarian Times* August 1997: 70-71.

Murray, M.T., N.D. *The Healing Power of Herbs.* Rocklin, Calif.: Prima Publishing, 1992.

APPENDIX B

Recommended Reading for General Health

Blumenthal, M. *The Complete German Commission E Monographs.* Austin, Texas: American Botanical Council in cooperation with Integrative Medicine Communications, 1998.

Brown, D.J., N.D. *Herbal Prescriptions for Better Health.* Rocklin, Calif.: Prima Publishing, 1996.

Buckle, J., R.N., MA., Cert. Ed. *Clinical Aromatherapy in Nursing.* Arnold, London. 1997.

Dossey, L., M.D. *Healing Words.* San Francisco: Harper San Francisco, 1993.

Duke, J.A., Ph.D., *Herbs of the Bible.* Loveland, Colo.: Interweave Press, 1999.

Duke, J.A., Ph.D., *The Green Pharmacy.* Emmaus, Penn.: Rodale Press, 1997.

Erasmus, U. *Fats that Heal, Fats that Kill.* Burnaby, British Columbia: Alive Books, 1999.

Gladstar, R. *Herbal Healing for Women.* New York: Fireside, 1993.

Gleick, J. *Chaos: Making a New Science.* New York: Penguin, 1988.

Grieve, Mrs. M., *A Modern Herbal-Vols. 1&2.* New York: Dover Publications,1971.

Hobbs, C., L.Ac., *Medicinal Mushrooms.* Santa Cruz, Calif.: Botanica Press,1986.

Keuneke, R. *Total Breast Health.* New York: Kensington Books, 1998.

Leung, A. Y. and and S. Foster *Encyclopedia of Common Natural Ingredients* New York: John Wiley & Sons, Inc., 1996.

Murray, M., N.D. and J. Pizzorno, N.D., *Encyclopedia of Natural Medicine.* Rocklin, Calif.: Prima Publishing, 1991.

Pizzorno, J.E., N.D., and M. Murray, N.D., *Textbook of Natural Medicine* (2ⁿᵈ edition). London: Churchill Livingstone / Harcourt Brace and Company Limited,1999.

Weatherby, C. and Leonid Gordin, M.D. *The Arthritis Bible.* Rochester, Vermont: Healing Arts Press,1999.

Weil, A., M.D., *Spontaneous Healing.* New York: Alfred A. Knopf, Inc., 1995. *8 Weeks to Optimum Health.* Fawcett Books, 1998.

Yance, D. and A. Valentine *Herbal Medicine, Healing and Cancer.* New Canaan, Conn.: Keats Publishing, 1999.

REFERENCES

We have attempted to identify all of the primary scientific materials on which we relied, organized under each book chapter by date of publication. To simplify access to these materials, we have followed the exact citation form used for Medline (PubMed) scientific references by the Library of Medicine. To further facilitate review of the scientific papers, we have, where available, set forth at the end of the citation the PMID number that can be used to retrieve the study from PubMed.

Chapter One: Arthritis—From NSAIDS to the "Safe Aspirin"

Rheum Dis Clin North Am 1999 May;25(2):359-78 Selective cyclooxygenase-2 inhibitors. Golden BD, Abramson SB Department of Rheumatology, Hospital for Joint Diseases, New York, New York, USA. PMID 10356423

Chapter Two: Understanding Inflammation and Balance

Lancet 1999 Dec;354:2106-2111 Celecoxib associated with fewer GI side effects than diclofenac (reported online at: www.reutershealth.com)

PSL Group – Press Release Dec 15, 1999 FDA Committee Recommends Approval of Celebrex for Familial Adenomatous Polyposis. (reported online at: http://www.pslgroup.com)

JAMA 1999, Nov. 24, Vol 282, No. 20 Vioxx, For AO Symptoms, Has Few GI Problems When Compared To NSAIDS. (reported online at: www.pslgroup.com)

Gastroentology 1999 Oct Vioxx Causes Fewer Endoscopic Ulcers Than Ibuprofen, Study Shows. (reported online at: http://www.pslgroup.com)

PSL Group – Press Release 1999 Oct APS: Celebrex Provides Relief From Post-Operative Pain. (presented at the annual meeting of the American Pain Society; reported online at: http://www.pslgroup.com)

Obstetrics and Gynecology 1999 Oct Osteoarthritis Drug, Vioxx, Relieves Menstrual Pain. (reported online at: www.pslgroup.com)

Ann Pharmacother 1999 Sep;33(9):979-88 The cyclooxygenase-2 inhibitors: safety and effectiveness. Kaplan-Machlis B, Klostermeyer BS Department of Clinical Pharmacy, School of Pharmacy, Robert C Byrd Health Sciences Center of West Virginia University, Charleston 25304, USA. bkaplan@wvu.edu PMID 10492503

J Am Geriatr Soc 1999 Aug;47(8):1016-25 Emerging evidence for inflammation in conditions frequently affecting older adults: report of a symposium. Hamerman D, Berman JW, Albers GW, Brown DL, Silver D PMID: 10443865, UI: 99371465

Clin Ther 1999 Jul;21(7):1131-57 Selective cyclooxygenase-2 inhibitors for the treatment of arthritis. Fung HB, Kirschenbaum HL Arnold & Marie Schwartz College of Pharmacy and Health Sciences, Long Island University, Brooklyn, New York 11201, USA. PMID 10463513

Osteoarthritis Cartilage 1999 Jul;7(4):406-8 COX-2 in synovial tissues. Crofford LJ Division of Rheumatology, University of Michigan, 5510E MSRB I, 1150 W. Medical Center Dr., Ann Arbor,MI PMID 10419782

J Am Osteopath Assoc 1999 Jun;99(6):322-5 Specific cyclooxygenase-2 (COX-2) inhibitors. Rubin BR Department of Internal Medicine, University of North Texas Health Science Center, Fort Worth/Texas College of Osteopathic Medicine 76107, USA. brubin@hsc.unt.edu PMID 10405519

Int J Biochem Cell Biol 1999 May;31(5):551-7 Cyclooxygenase-1 and -2 isoenzymes. Hla T, Bishop-Bailey D, Liu CH, Schaefers HJ, Trifan OC. Department of Physiology, School of Medicine, University of Connecticut Health Center, Farmington 06030, USA. hla@sun.uchc.edu PMID 10399316

Inflamm Res 1999 May;48(5):247-54 Clinical experience with cyclooxygenase-2 inhibitors. van Ryn J, Pairet M Department of Pulmonary Research, Boehringer Ingelheim Pharma KG, Biberach an der Riss, Germany. joanne.vanryn@bc.boehringer-ingelheim.com PMID 10391112

Am J Med 1999 May 31;106(5B):43S-50S Cyclooxygenase-2 specificity and its clinical implications. Lefkowith JB Research and Development, G.D. Searle and Company, Research and Development, Chicago, Illinois 60077, USA. PMID 10390127

Am J Med 1999 May 31;106(5B):37S-42S Role and regulation of cyclooxygenase-2 during inflammation. Simon LS Department of Medicine, Harvard Medical School of Medicine, Beth Israel Deaconess Medical Center, Boston, Massachusetts 02215, USA. PMID 10390126

Rheum Dis Clin North Am 1999 May;25(2):359-78 Selective cyclooxygenase-2 inhibitors. Golden BD, Abramson SB Department of Rheumatology, Hospital for Joint Diseases, New York, New York, USA. PMID 10356423

Cleve Clin J Med 1999 May;66(5):285-92 COX 2-selective NSAIDs: biology, promises, and concerns. Mandell BF Department of Rheumatic and Immunologic Diseases, Cleveland Clinic Foundation, OH 44195, USA. mandelb@ccf.org PMID 10330781

J Rheumatol 1999 Apr;26 Suppl 56:11-7 The evolution of arthritis antiinflammatory care: where are we today? Simon LS Beth Israel Deaconess Hospital, Harvard Medical School, Boston, Massachusetts, USA. PMID 10225535

Am J Orthop 1999 Mar;28(3 Suppl):13-8 Celecoxib, a COX-2—specific inhibitor: the clinical data. Fort J Medical Affairs, G.D. Searle & Co, Skokie, Illinois, USA. PMID 10193998

FASEB J 1999 Feb;13(2):245-51 Synergy between cyclo-oxygenase-2 induction and arachidonic acid supply in vivo: consequences for nonsteroidal antiinflammatory drug efficacy. Hamilton LC, Mitchell JA, Tomlinson AM, Warner TD Vascular Inflammation, The William Harvey Research Institute, Bartholomew's and the Royal School of Medicine and Dentistry, London, UK. PMID 9973312

J Rheumatol 1998 Dec;25(12):2298-303 The classification of cyclooxygenase inhibitors. Lipsky LP, Abramson SB, Crofford L, Dubois RN, Simon LS, van de Putte LB PMID 9858421

FASEB J 1998 Sep;12(12):1063-73 Cyclooxygenase in biology and disease. Dubois RN, Abramson SB, Crofford L, Gupta RA, Simon LS, Van De Putte LB, Lipsky PE Department of Medicine/GI, Vanderbilt University Medical Center, Nashville, Tennessee 37232-2279, USA. duboisrn@ctrvax.vanderbilt edu PMID 9737710

Ned Tijdschr Geneeskd 1998 Aug 1;142(31):1762-5 [Non-steroidal anti-inflammatory agents (NSAID's) with lesser side effects by selective inhibition of cyclo-oxygenase-2]. Bijlsma JW, Van de Putte LB Academisch Ziekenhuis, afd. Reumatologie en Klinische Immunologie, Utrecht. PMID 9856140

J Rheumatol Suppl 1998 May;51:2-7 Scientific rationale for specific inhibition of COX-2. Bolten WW Rheumaklinik Wiesbaden II, Germany. PMID 9596548

Am J Med 1998 Mar 30;104(3A):2S-8S; discussion 21S-22S Mechanism of action of nonsteroidal anti-inflammatory drugs. Vane JR, Botting RM The William Harvey Research Institute, St Bartholomew's Hospital Medical College, London, United Kingdom. PMID 9572314

J Rheumatol 1997 Jul;24 Suppl 49:20-4 Pain management in osteoarthritis: the role of COX-2 inhibitors. Lane NE Department of Medicine, University of California at San Francisco 94143, USA. nelane@itsa.ucsf.edu PMID 9249647

J Rheumatol 1997 Jul;24 Suppl 49:9-14 Outcome of specific COX-2 inhibition in rheumatoid arthritis. Lipsky PE, Isakson PC Department of Internal Medicine, University of Texas Southwestern Medical Center, Dallas 75235-8884, USA. PMID 9249645

Ital J Gastroenterol 1996 Dec;28 Suppl 4:28-9 New NSAIDs and gastroduodenal damage. Folco GC Istituto di Scienze Farmacologiche, Universita di Milano, Italy. PMID 9032579

Gastroenterol Clin North Am 1996 Jun;25(2):363-72 Cyclooxygenase-2 inhibitors: a new class of anti-inflammatory agents that spare the gastrointestinal tract. Masferrer JL, Isakson PC, Seibert K Inflammatory Diseases Research, G.D. Searle at Monsanto Corporation, St. Louis, Missouri, USA. PMID 9229578

Ginger: Common Spice and Wonder Drug Schulick, P., Brattleboro, VT; Herbal Free Press 1996

Chapter Three: COX-2 Extends to the World of Cancer

Gut 1999 Nov;45(5):730-2 Differential expression of cyclooxygenase 2 in human colorectal cancer. Dimberg J, Samuelsson A, Hugander A, Soderkvist P. Department of Biomedicine and Surgery, Division of Cell Biology, Faculty of Health Sciences, Linkoping, Sweden. PMID 10517910

Eur Respir J 1999 Aug;14(2):412-8 Expression and localization of cyclo-oxygenase isoforms in non-small cell lung cancer. Watkins DN, Lenzo JC, Segal A, Garlepp MJ, Thompson PJ. Asthma and Allergy Research Unit, The University Dept of Medicine, Queen Elizabeth II Medical Centre, Nedlands, Western Australia, Australia. PMID 10515422

Recent Results Cancer Res 1999;151:45-67 Metabolic targets of cancer chemoprevention: interruption of tumor development by inhibitors of arachidonic acid metabolism. Marks F, Furstenberger G, Muller-Decker K German Cancer Research Center, Heidelberg, Germany PMID 10337718

Am J Med 1998 Nov 2;105(5A):44S-52S Future trends in the development of safer nonsteroidal anti-inflammatory drugs. Wolfe MM Department of Medicine, Boston University School of Medicine, Massachusetts 02118, USA. PMID 9855176

J Assoc Acad Minor Phys 1998;9(2):40-4 Use and safety of aspirin in the chemoprevention of colorectal cancer. Singh AK, Trotman BW. Department of Medicine, UMDNJ-University Hospital, Newark, New Jersey 07103-2714, USA. PMID 9648425

Chapter Four: The Intimacies Between COX-2 and Cancer

Semin Oncol 1999 Oct;26(5):499-504 Chemoprevention of colorectal cancer through inhibition of cyclooxygenase-2. Dannenberg AJ, Zakim D Department of Medicine, The New York Hospital-Cornell Medical Center and Strang Cancer Prevention Center, NY 10021, USA. PMID 10528897

Thromb Res 1999 Aug 15;95(4):155-61 Inhibition of smoking-induced platelet aggregation by aspirin and pycnogenol. Putter M, Grotemeyer KH, Wurthwein G, Araghi-Niknam M, Watson RR, Hosseini S, Rohdewald P Department of Neurology, Westfalische Wilhelms-Universitat Munster, Germany. PMID 10498385

Biomed Pharmacother 1999 Aug;53(7):303-8 The prevention of colorectal cancer by aspirin use. Giovannucci E Department of Medicine, Brigham and Women's Hospital, Boston, MA 02115, USA. PMID 10472428

J Am Geriatr Soc 1999 Aug;47(8):1016-25 Emerging evidence for inflammation in conditions frequently affecting older adults: report of a symposium. Hamerman D, Berman JW, Albers GW, Brown DL, Silver D PMID: 10443865, UI: 99371465

Int J Biochem Cell Biol 1999 May;31(5):551-7 Cyclooxygenase-1 and -2 isoenzymes. Hla T, Bishop-Bailey D, Liu CH, Schaefers HJ, Trifan OC Department of Physiology, School of Medicine, University of Connecticut Health Center, Farmington 06030, USA. hla@sun.uchc.edu PMID 10399316

Cancer Res 1999 Mar 1;59(5):987-90 Cyclooxygenase-2 expression is up-regulated in human pancreatic cancer. Tucker ON, Dannenberg AJ, Yang EK, Zhang F, Teng L, Daly JM, Soslow RA, Masferrer JL, Woerner BM, Koki AT, Fahey TJ 3rd Department of Surgery, New York Presbyterian Hospital and Weill Medical College of Cornell University, New York, New York 10021, USA. PMID 10070951

Medscape Womens Health 1999 Jan-Feb;4(1):4 Hormone alterations in breast cancer: examining the hypotheses. Hindle WH University of Southern California School of Medicine, Los Angeles, USA. PMID 10089557

Int J Mol Med 1998 Dec;2(6):715-9 Cox-2, iNOS and p53 as play-makers of tumor angiogenesis (review). Chiarugi V, Magnelli L, Gallo O Laboratory of Molecular Biology, Institute of General Pathology, Firenze, Italy. PMID 9850741

J Natl Cancer Inst 1998 Nov 4;90(21):1609-20 Cyclooxygenase-2 inhibitors in tumorigenesis (Part II). Taketo MM Laboratory of Biomedical Genetics, Graduate School of Pharmaceutical Sciences, University of Tokyo, Bunkyo, Japan.

J Natl Cancer Inst 1998 Oct 21;90(20):1529-36 Cyclooxygenase-2 inhibitors in tumorigenesis (part I). Taketo MM Laboratory of Biomedical Genetics, Graduate School of Pharmaceutical Sciences, University of Tokyo, Bunkyo, Japan. taketo@mol.f.u-tokyo.ac.jp PMID 9811310

Cancer Res 1998 Jun 1;58(11):2323-7 Antioxidants reduce cyclooxygenase-2 expression, prostaglandin production, and proliferation in colorectal cancer cells. Chinery R, Beauchamp RD, Shyr Y, Kirkland SC, Coffey RJ, Morrow JD Department of Medicine, The Vanderbilt Cancer Center, Vanderbilt University Medical Center, Nashville, Tennessee 37232, USA. PMID 9622066

Cell 1998 May 29;93(5):705-16 Published erratum appears in Cell 1998 Jul 24;94(2):following 271 Cyclooxygenase regulates angiogenesis induced by colon cancer cells. Tsujii M, Kawano S, Tsuji S, Sawaoka H, Hori M, DuBois RN Department of Medicine, Vanderbilt University Medical Center, VA Medical Center, Nashville, Tennessee 37232, USA. PMID 9630216

Histol Histopathol 1998 Apr;13(2):591-7 Chemopreventive effects of NSAIDs against colorectal cancer: regulation of apoptosis and mitosis by COX-1 and COX-2. Watson AJ Department of Medicine, Hope Hospital, University of Manchester, Salford, UK. PMID 9589912

J Clin Gastroenterol 1998;27 Suppl 1:S1-11 Prostaglandins in the stomach: an update. Arakawa T, Higuchi K, Fukuda T, Fujiwara Y, Kobayashi K, Kuroki T Third Department of Internal Medicine, Osaka City University Medical School, Osaka, Japan. PMID 9872492

Proc Soc Exp Biol Med 1997 Nov;216(2):201-10 Inhibition of cyclooxygenase: a novel approach to cancer prevention. Subbaramaiah K, Zakim D, Weksler BB, Dannenberg AJ Department of Medicine, The New York Hospital-Cornell Medical Center, New York 10021, USA. PMID 9349689

Chapter Five: A Refocus on the Safety of Celebrex and Vioxx

PSL Group – Press Release 1999 Dec FDA Committee Recommends Approval of Celebrex for Familial Adenomatous Polyposis www.pslgroup.com

J Rheumatol 1999 Apr;26 Suppl 56:25-30 Specific COX-2 inhibitors in arthritis, oncology, and beyond: where is the science headed? Lipsky PE Department of Internal Medicine, The University of Texas Southwestern Medical Center at Dallas, 75235-8884, USA. PMID 10225537

J Rheumatol 1999 Apr;26 Suppl 56:25-30 Specific COX-2 inhibitors in arthritis, oncology, and beyond: where is the science headed? Lipsky PE PMID: 10225537, UI: 99240067

Annu Rev Pharmacol Toxicol 1998;38:97-120 Cyclooxygenases 1 and 2. Vane JR, Bakhle YS, Botting RM William Harvey Research Institute, St Bartholomew's, London, United Kingdom. PMID 9597150

MedscapeWire 1999 Jan How Super are the 'Super Aspirins"? – New Cox-2 Inhibitors May Elevate Cardiovascular Risk. University of Pennsylvania Medical Center www.medscape.com)

Chapter Six: The Confluence of Science and Traditional Medicine

USDA Phytochemical Database www.ars-grin.gov/duke/

NAPRALERT Database, University of Illinois. For information, contact: quinn@pcog1.pmmp.uic.edu

Chapter Seven: Green Tea

J Cancer Res Clin Oncol 1999 Nov;125(11):589-97 Two stages of cancer prevention with green tea. Fujiki, H PMID 10541965

Carcinogenesis 1999 Oct;20(10):1945-52 Suppression of inducible cyclooxygenase and inducible nitric oxide synthase by apigenin and related flavonoids in mouse macrophages. Liang YC, Huang YT, Tsai SH, Lin-Shiau SY, Chen CF, Lin JK Institute of Biochemistry, College of Medicine, National Taiwan University, No. 1, Section 1, Taipei, Taiwan. PMID 10506109

Altern Med Rev 1999 Oct;4(5):360-70 Green tea (Camellia sinensis) extract and its possible role in the prevention of cancer. Brown MD Sage Health Clinic, Bend, OR, USA. drcowboyup@hotmail.com PMID 10559550

Mutat Res 1999 Jul 16;428(1-2):339-44 Green tea and cancer chemoprevention. Suganuma M, Okabe S, Sueoka N, Sueoka E, Matsuyama S, Imai K, Nakachi K, Fujiki H Saitama Cancer Center Research Institute, Ina, Kitaadachi-gun, Saitama 362-0806, Japan. PMID 10518005

Mutat Res 1999 Jul 16;428(1-2):305-27 Molecular mechanisms of chemopreventive effects of selected dietary and medicinal phenolic substances. Surh Y Laboratory of Biochemistry and Molecular Toxicology, College of Pharmacy, Seoul National University, Shinlim-dong, Kwanak-gu, Seoul, South Korea. surh@plaza.snu.ac.kr PMID 10518003

Cancer Lett 1999 Jul 1;141(1-2):159-65 Anti-metastatic activity of curcumin and catechin. Menon LG, Kuttan R, Kuttan G Amala Cancer Research Centre, Trichur, India. PMID 10454257

Semin Urol Oncol 1999 May;17(2):70-6 Prostate cancer chemoprevention by green tea. Gupta S, Ahmad N, Mukhtar H Department of Dermatology, University Hospitals of Cleveland, Case Western Reserve University, OH 44106, USA. PMID 10332919

Proc Natl Acad Sci U S A 1999 Apr 13;96(8):4524-9 Prevention of collagen-induced arthritis in mice by a polyphenolic fraction from green tea. Haqqi TM, Anthony DD, Gupta S, Ahmad N, Lee MS, Kumar GK, Mukhtar H Department of Medicine, Division of Rheumatic Diseases, Case Western Reserve University, 10900 Euclid Avenue, Cleveland, OH 44106, USA. PMID 10200295

Proc Soc Exp Biol Med 1999 Apr;220(4):229-33 Inhibitory effect of green and black tea on tumor growth. Conney AH, Lu Y, Lou Y, Xie J, Huang M Laboratory for Cancer Research, Department of Chemical Biology, College of Pharmacy, Rutgers, The State University of New Jersey, Piscataway, New Jersey 08854-8020, USA. PMID 10202394

Proc Soc Exp Biol Med 1999 Apr;220(4):225-8 Mechanistic findings of green tea as cancer preventive for humans. Fujiki H, Suganuma M, Okabe S, Sueoka E, Suga K, Imai K, Nakachi K, Kimura S Saitama Cancer Center Research Institute, Ina, Kitaadachi-gun, Saitama 362-0806, Japan. hfuji@saitama-cc.go.jp PMID 10202393

Proc Natl Acad Sci U S A 1999 Apr 13;96(8):4524-9 Prevention of collagen-induced arthritis in mice by a polyphenolic fraction from green tea. Haqqi TM, Anthony DD, Gupta S, Ahmad N, Lee MS, Kumar GK, Mukhtar H Department of Medicine, Division of Rheumatic Diseases, Case Western Reserve University, 10900 Euclid Avenue, Cleveland, OH 44106, USA. PMID 10200295

Photochem Photobiol 1999 Feb;69(2):148-53 Polyphenolic antioxidant (-)-epigallocatechin-3-gallate from green tea reduces UVB-induced inflammatory responses and infiltration of leukocytes in human skin. Katiyar SK, Matsui MS, Elmets CA, Mukhtar H Department of Dermatology, Case Western Reserve University, Cleveland, OH 44106, USA. PMID 10048310

Cancer Res 1999 Jan 1;59(1):44-7 Synergistic effects of (—)-epigallocatechin gallate with (—)-epicatechin, sulindac, or tamoxifen on cancer-preventive activity in the human lung cancer cell line PC-9. Suganuma M, Okabe S, Kai Y, Sueoka N, Sueoka E, Fujiki H Saitama Cancer Center Research Institute, Japan. PMID 9892181

J Nutr 1998 Dec;128(12):2334-40 Green tea polyphenols block endotoxin-induced tumor necrosis factor-production and lethality in a murine model. Yang F, de Villiers WJ, McClain CJ, Varilek GW Graduate Program in Nutritional Sciences, Department of Internal Medicine, University of Kentucky, Lexington, KY 40536, USA. PMID 9868178

Inflamm Res 1998 Oct;47 Suppl 2:S78-87 Anti-inflammatory drugs and their mechanism of action. Vane JR, Botting RM The William Harvey Research Institute, St. Bartholomew's and the Royal London School of Medicine and Dentistry, Queen Mary and Westfield College, UK. PMID 9831328

Biochem J 1998 Sep 15;334 (Pt 3):577-84 An array of binding sites for hepatocyte nuclear factor 4 of high and low affinities modulates the liver-specific enhancer for the human alpha1-microglobulin/bikunin precursor. Rouet P, Raguenez G, Ruminy P, Salier JP INSERM Unit-78 and Institut Federatif de Recherches Multidisciplinaires sur les Peptides, Faculte de Medecine-Pharmacie, 22 Boulevard Gambetta, 76000 Rouen, France. PMID 9719465

Biochem Biophys Res Commun 1998 Aug 19;249(2):391-6 Telomerase inhibition, telomere shortening, and senescence of cancer cells by tea catechins. Naasani I, Seimiya H, Tsuruo T Cancer Chemotherapy Center, Japanese Foundation for Cancer Research, Kami-Ikebukuro, Tokyo, Toshima-ku, 170-8455, Japan. inaasani@ns.jfcr.or.jp PMID 9712707

Cancer Lett 1998 Aug 14;130(1-2):1-7 Induction of apoptosis in prostate cancer cell lines by the green tea component, (-)-epigallocatechin-3-gallate. Paschka AG, Butler R, Young CY Department of Urology, Mayo Clinic/Foundation, Rochester, MN 55905, USA. PMID 9751250

Planta Med 1998 Aug;64(6):520-4 Flavan-3-ols isolated from some medicinal plants inhibiting COX-1 and COX-2 catalysed prostaglandin biosynthesis. Noreen Y, Serrano G, Perera P, Bohlin L Department of Pharmacy, Uppsala University, Sweden.

Exp Lung Res 1998 Jul-Aug;24(4):629-39 Tea and tea polyphenols inhibit cell hyperproliferation, lung tumorigenesis, and tumor progression. Yang CS, Yang GY, Landau JM, Kim S, Liao J Laboratory for Cancer Research, College of Pharmacy, Rutgers University, Piscataway, New Jersey, USA. PMID 9659588

Mutat Res 1998 Jun 18;402(1-2):307-10 Cancer inhibition by green tea. Fujiki H, Suganuma M, Okabe S, Sueoka N, Komori A, Sueoka E, Kozu T, Tada Y, Suga K, Imai K, Nakachi K Saitama Cancer Center Research Institute, Ina, Kitaadachi-gun, Saitama 362, Japan. PMID 9675322

Carcinogenesis 1998 Apr;19(4):611-6 Inhibition of growth and induction of apoptosis in human cancer cell lines by tea polyphenols. Yang GY, Liao J, Kim K, Yurkow EJ, Yang CS Laboratory for Cancer Research, College of Pharmacy, Rutgers University, Piscataway, NJ 08855-0789, USA. PMID 9600345

Oncol Rep 1998 Mar-Apr;5(2):527-9 Induction of apoptosis in human stomach cancer cells by green tea catechins. Hibasami H, Komiya T, Achiwa Y, Ohnishi K, Kojima T, Nakanishi K, Akashi K, Hara Y Faculty of Medicine, Mie University, Tsu-city, Mie 514, Japan. PMID 9468594

Jpn J Cancer Res 1998 Mar;89(3):254-61 Influence of drinking green tea on breast cancer malignancy among Japanese patients. Nakachi K, Suemasu K, Suga K, Takeo T, Imai K, Higashi Y Department of Epidemiology, Saitama Cancer Center Research Institute. PMID 9600118

Carcinogenesis 1998 Mar;19(3):419-24 Quantitation of chemopreventive synergism between (-)-epigallocatechin-3-gallate and curcumin in normal, premalignant and malignant human oral epithelial cells. Khafif A, Schantz SP, Chou TC, Edelstein D, Sacks PG Department of Surgery, Head and Neck Surgery, Memorial Sloan-Kettering Cancer Center, New York, NY 10021, USA. PMID 9525275

J Nat Prod 1998 Jan;61(1):8-12 Two new isoflavones from Ceiba pentandra and their effect on cyclooxygenase-catalyzed prostaglandin biosynthesis. Noreen Y, el-Seedi H, Perera P, Bohlin L Department of Pharmacy, Uppsala University, Sweden.

J Nat Prod 1998 Jan;61(1):2-7 Development of a radiochemical cyclooxygenase-1 and -2 in vitro assay for identification of natural products as inhibitors of prostaglandin biosynthesis. Noreen Y, Ringbom T, Perera P, Danielson H, Bohlin L Department of Pharmacy, Uppsala University, Sweden. PMID 9741297, 9461647, 9461646

Life Sci 1998;63(16):1397-403 Growth inhibition of leukemic cells by (-)-epigallocatechin gallate, the main constituent of green tea. Otsuka T, Ogo T, Eto T, Asano Y, Suganuma M, Niho Y First Department of Internal Medicine, Faculty of Medicine, Kyushu University, Fukuoka, Japan. PMID 9952285

Adv Exp Med Biol 1998;439:237-48 Inhibition of neoplastic transformation and bioavailability of dietary flavonoid agents. Franke AA, Cooney RV, Custer LJ, Mordan LJ, Tanaka Y Cancer Research Center of Hawaii, Honolulu 96813, USA. PMID 9781307

J Natl Cancer Inst 1997 Dec 17;89(24):1881-6 Green tea constituent epigallocatechin-3-gallate and induction of apoptosis and cell cycle arrest in human carcinoma cells. Ahmad N, Feyes DK, Nieminen AL, Agarwal R, Mukhtar H Department of Dermatology, School of Medicine, Case Western Reserve University, Cleveland, OH 44106, USA. PMID 9414176

Biochem Pharmacol 1997 Dec 15;54(12):1281-6 Inhibition of inducible nitric oxide synthase gene expression and enzyme activity by epigallocatechin gallate, a natural product from green tea. Chan MM, Fong D, Ho CT, Huang HI Department of Biomedical Sciences, Pennsylvania College of Podiatric Medicine, Philadelphia 19107-2496, USA. chan@biology.rutgers.edu PMID 9393670

Biosci Biotechnol Biochem 1997 Sep;61(9):1504-6 Inhibition of collagenases from mouse lung carcinoma cells by green tea catechins and black tea theaflavins. Sazuka M, Imazawa H, Shoji Y, Mita T, Hara Y, Isemura M School of Food and Nutritional Sciences, University of Shizuoka, Japan. PMID 9339552

Jpn J Cancer Res 1997 Jul;88(7):639-43 Mechanisms of growth inhibition of human lung cancer cell line, PC-9, by tea polyphenols. Okabe S, Suganuma M, Hayashi M, Sueoka E, Komori A, Fujiki H Saitama Cancer Center Research Institute. PMID 9310136

Mol Pharmacol 1997 Jun;51(6):907-12 Sodium salicylate inhibits cyclo-oxygenase-2 activity independently of transcription factor (nuclear factor kappaB) activation: role of arachidonic acid. Mitchell JA, Saunders M, Barnes PJ, Newton R, Belvisi MG Department of Anaesthesia and Critical Care Medicine, The Royal Brompton Hospital, London, England. j.mitchell@rbh.nthames.nhs.uk PMID 9187256

J Cell Biochem Suppl 1997;27:52-8 Influence of tea catechins on the digestive tract. Hara Y Food Research Institute, Mitsui Norin Co., Ltd., Shizuoka Pref., Japan. PMID 9591193

Jpn J Cancer Res 1996 Oct;87(10):1034-8 Inhibitory effects of tea catechins, black tea extract and oolong tea extract on hepatocarcinogenesis in rat. Matsumoto N, Kohri T, Okushio K, Hara Y Food Research Laboratories, Mitsui Norin Co., Ltd., Shizuoka, Japan. PMID 8957060

Fukuoka Igaku Zasshi 1996 Oct;87(10):215-21 [(-)-Epigallocatechin gallate, the main constituent of Japanese green tea, inhibits tumor promotion of okadaic acid]. Yoshizawa S First Department of Internal Medicine, Faculty of Medicine, Kyushu University, Fukuoka. PMID 8940799

Cancer Res 1996 Aug 15;56(16):3711-5 A new process of cancer prevention mediated through inhibition of tumor necrosis factor alpha expression. Suganuma M, Okabe S, Sueoka E, Iida N, Komori A, Kim SJ, Fujiki H Saitama Cancer Center Research Institute, Japan. PMID 8706012

Cancer 1996 Apr 15;77(8 Suppl):1662-7 Inhibitory effects and toxicity of green tea polyphenols for gastrointestinal carcinogenesis. Yamane T, Nakatani H, Kikuoka N, Matsumoto H, Iwata Y, Kitao Y, Oya K, Takahashi T First Department of Surgery, Kyoto Prefectural University of Medicine, Japan. PMID 8608559

Photochem Photobiol 1995 Nov;62(5):855-61 Protection against ultraviolet-B radiation-induced local and systemic suppression of contact hypersensitivity and edema responses in C3H/HeN mice by green tea polyphenols. Katiyar SK, Elmets CA, Agarwal R, Mukhtar H Department of Dermatology, University Hospitals of Cleveland, Case Western Reserve University, OH 44106, USA. PMID 8570723

Cancer Lett 1995 Sep 25;96(2):239-43 Growth inhibition and regression of human prostate and breast tumors in athymic mice by tea epigallocatechin gallate. Liao S, Umekita Y, Guo J, Kokontis JM, Hiipakka RA Ben May Institute, Department of Biochemistry and Molecular Biology, University of Chicago, IL 60637, USA. PMID 7585463

J Pharmacol Exp Ther 1995 Aug;274(2):602-8 Ameliorative effects of tea catechins on active oxygen-related nerve cell injuries. Matsuoka Y, Hasegawa H, Okuda S, Muraki T, Uruno T, Kubota K Department of Pharmacology, Faculty of Pharmaceutical Sciences, Science University of Tokyo, Japan. PMID 7636719

J Ethnopharmacol 1995 Jun;46(3):167-74 Anti-ulcer effect of the hot water extract of black tea (Camellia sinensis). Maity S, Vedasiromoni JR, Ganguly DK Division of Pharmacology and Experimental Therapeutics, Indian Institute of Chemical Biology, Jadavpur, Calcutta. PMID 7564415

Cancer Lett 1994 Aug 15;83(1-2):143-7 Prevention of heterocyclic amine formation by tea and tea polyphenols. Weisburger JH, Nagao M, Wakabayashi K, Oguri A American Health Foundation, Valhalla, NY 10595-1599. PMID 8062207

Cancer Detect Prev 1994;18(1):1-7 A new tumor promotion pathway and its inhibitors. Fujiki H, Suganuma M, Komori A, Yatsunami J, Okabe S, Ohta T, Sueoka E Cancer Prevention Division, National Cancer Center Research Institute, Tokyo, Japan. PMID 8162603

Fortschr Med 1993 Nov 30;111(33):530-2 [Antiphlogistic effect of salicylic acid and its derivatives]. Binder M, Zeiller P Luitpold Pharma GmbH, Munchen. PMID 8307537

Photochem Photobiol 1993 Nov;58(5):695-700 Protection against ultraviolet B radiation-induced effects in the skin of SKH-1 hairless mice by a polyphenolic fraction isolated from green tea. Agarwal R, Katiyar SK, Khan SG, Mukhtar H Department of Dermatology, University Hospitals of Cleveland, OH. PMID 8284325

Jpn J Clin Oncol 1993 Jun;23(3):186-90 Anticarcinogenic activity of green tea polyphenols. Komori A, Yatsunami J, Okabe S, Abe S, Hara K, Suganuma M, Kim SJ, Fujiki H Cancer Prevention Division, National Cancer Center Research Institute, Tokyo. PMID 8350491

Carcinogenesis 1993 Mar;14(3):361-5 Protection against 12-O-tetradecanoylphorbol-13-acetate-caused inflammation in SENCAR mouse ear skin by polyphenolic fraction isolated from green tea. Katiyar SK, Agarwal R, Ekker S, Wood GS, Mukhtar H Department of Dermatology, University Hospitals of Cleveland, Case Western Reserve University, OH. PMID 8453711

Cancer Res 1992 Dec 15;52(24):6890-7 Inhibition of 12-O-tetradecanoylphorbol-13-acetate-caused tumor promotion in 7,12-dimethylbenz[a]anthracene initiated SENCAR mouse skin by a polyphenolic fraction isolated from green tea. Katiyar SK, Agarwal R, Wood GS, Mukhtar H Department of Dermatology, University Hospitals of Cleveland, Case Western Reserve University, Ohio. PMID 1458478

Prev Med 1992 Jul;21(4):510-9 Chemopreventive effects of green tea components on hepatic carcinogenesis. Klaunig JE Department of Pharmacology and Toxicology, Indiana University School of Medicine, Indianapolis 46202. PMID 1409492

Prev Med 1992 Jul;21(4):503-9 Anticarcinogenic effects of (-)-epigallocatechin gallate. Fujiki H, Yoshizawa S, Horiuchi T, Suganuma M, Yatsunami J, Nishiwaki S, Okabe S, Nishiwaki-Matsushima R, Okuda T, Sugimura T Cancer Prevention Division, National Cancer Center Research Institute, Tokyo, Japan. PMID 1409491

Carcinogenesis 1992 Jun;13(6):947-54 Inhibitory effect of topical application of a green tea polyphenol fraction on tumor initiation and promotion in mouse skin. Huang MT, Ho CT, Wang ZY, Ferraro T, Finnegan-Olive T, Lou YR, Mitchell JM, Laskin JD, Newmark H, Yang CS, et al Department of Chemical Biology and Pharmacognosy, College of Pharmacy, Rutgers, State University of New Jersey, Piscataway 08855-0789. PMID 1600615

Chin Med Sci J 1991 Dec;6(4):233-8 Progress in studies on the antimutagenicity and anticarcinogenicity of green tea epicatechins. Cheng S, Ding L, Zhen Y, Lin P, Zhu Y, Chen Y, Hu X Institute of Oncology, CAMS, Beijing. PMID 1813062

Clin Exp Metastasis 1991 Jan-Feb;9(1):13-25 Effect of catechins and citrus flavonoids on invasion in vitro. Bracke M, Vyncke B, Opdenakker G, Foidart JM, De Pestel G, Mareel M Department of Radiotherapy and Nuclear Medicine, University Hospital, Gent, Belgium. PMID 1901781

Chung Kuo I Hsueh Ko Hsueh Yuan Hsueh Pao 1989 Aug;11(4):259-64 [Inhibitory effect of green tea extract on promotion and related action of TPA]. Cheng SJ PMID 2532970

Chapter Eight: Chinese Goldthread and Barberry

Carcinogenesis 1999 Oct;20(10):1945-52 Suppression of inducible cyclooxygenase and inducible nitric oxide synthase by apigenin and related flavonoids in mouse macrophages. Liang YC, Huang YT, Tsai SH, Lin-Shiau SY, Chen CF, Lin JK Institute of Biochemistry, College of Medicine, National Taiwan University, No. 1, Section 1, Taipei, Taiwan. PMID 10506109

J Ethnopharmacol 1999 Aug;66(2):227-33 Inhibition by berberine of cyclooxygenase-2 transcriptional activity in human colon cancer cells. Fukuda K, Hibiya Y, Mutoh M, Koshiji M, Akao S, Fujiwara H Department of Oriental Medicine, Gifu University School of Medicine, Japan. kfukuda@cc.gifu-u.ac.jp PMID 10433483

Planta Med 1999 May;65(4):381-3 Inhibition of activator protein 1 activity by berberine in human hepatoma cells. Fukuda K, Hibiya Y, Mutoh M, Koshiji M, Akao S, Fujiwara H PMID 10364850

Food Chem Toxicol 1999 Apr;37(4):319-26 Effects of berberine on arylamine N-acetyltransferase activity in human bladder tumour cells. Chung JG, Wu LT, Chu CB, Jan JY, Ho CC, Tsou MF, Lu HF, Chen GW, Lin JG, Wang TF Department of Microbiology, China Medical College, Taichung, Taiwan, Republic of China. PMID 10418949

Am J Chin Med 1999;27(2):265-75 Effects of berberine on arylamine N-acetyltransferase activity in human colon tumor cells. Lin JG, Chung JG, Wu LT, Chen GW, Chang HL, Wang TF Institute of Chinese Medical Science, China Medical College, Taichung, Taiwan. PMID 10467460

Biol Pharm Bull 1998 Aug;21(8):814-7 Inhibitory effect of Coptidis Rhizoma and Scutellariae Radix on azoxymethane-induced aberrant crypt foci formation in rat colon. Fukutake M, Yokota S, Kawamura H, Iizuka A, Amagaya S, Fukuda K, Komatsu Y Central Research Laboratories, Tsumura & Co., Ibaraki, Japan. PMID 9743248

Int J Immunopharmacol 1996 Oct;18(10):553-61 Study on the anti-inflammatory action of Berberis vulgaris root extract, alkaloid fractions and pure alkaloids. Ivanovska N, Philipov S Institute of Microbiology, Bulgarian Academy of Sciences, Sofia, Bulgaria. PMID 9080249

Cancer Lett 1995 Jul 13;93(2):193-200 Berberine complexes with DNA in the berberine-induced apoptosis in human leukemic HL-60 cells. Kuo CL, Chou CC, Yung BY Graduate Institute of Pharmacology, Yang Ming Medical College, Taiwan, ROC. PMID 7621428

Chin Med J (Engl) 1990 Aug;103(8):658-65 Laboratory studies of berberine used alone and in combination with 1,3-bis(2-chloroethyl)-1-nitrosourea to treat malignant brain tumors. Zhang RX, Dougherty DV, Rosenblum ML Department of Neurosurgery, Second Affiliated Hospital, Hebei Medical College, Shijiazhuang. PMID 2122945

Jpn J Pharmacol 1989 Mar;49(3):301-8 Features of the anti-ulcer effects of Orengedoku-to (a traditional Chinese medicine) and its component herb drugs. Takase H, Imanishi K, Miura O, Yumioka E, Watanabe H Kampo Research Laboratories, Kanebo Co., Ltd., Osaka, Japan. PMID 2747035

Oncology 1986;43(2):131-4 Berberine sulfate inhibits tumor-promoting activity of teleocidin in two-stage carcinogenesis on mouse skin. Nishino H, Kitagawa K, Fujiki H, Iwashima A PMID 3081844

Chapter Nine: Holy Basil*

J Ethnopharmacol 1999 Apr;65(1):13-9 Evaluation of the gastric antiulcer activity of fixed oil of Ocimum sanctum (Holy Basil). Singh S, Majumdar DK College of Pharmacy, University of Delhi, India. PMID 10350365

Oral Oncol 1999 Jan;35(1):112-9 Chemopreventive effect of Ocimum sanctum on DMBA-induced hamster buccal pouch carcinogenesis. Karthikeyan K, Ravichandran P, Govindasamy S Department of Biochemistry and Molecular Biology, University of Madras, India. PMID 10211319

Radiat Res 1999 Jan;151(1):74-8 In vivo radioprotection by ocimum flavonoids: survival of mice. Uma Devi P, Ganasoundari A, Rao BS, Srinivasan KK Department of Radiobiology, Kasturba Medical College, Manipal, India. PMID 9973087

Indian J Exp Biol 1998 Oct;36(10):1028-31 Comparative evaluation of antiinflammatory potential of fixed oil of different species of Ocimum and its possible mechanism of action. Singh S College of Pharmacy (University of Delhi), Pushp Vihar, India. PMID 10356964

J Nat Prod 1998 Oct;61(10):1212-5 Ursolic acid from Plantago major, a selective inhibitor of cyclooxygenase-2 catalyzed prostaglandin biosynthesis. Ringbom T, Segura L, Noreen Y, Perera P, Bohlin L Division of Pharmacognosy, Department of Pharmacy, Biomedical Centre, Uppsala University, Box 579, S-751 23 Uppsala, Sweden. PMID 9784154

Br J Radiol 1998 Jul;71(847):782-4 A comparative study of radioprotection by Ocimum flavonoids and synthetic aminothiol protectors in the mouse. Devi PU, Bisht KS, Vinitha M Department of Radiobiology, Kasturba Medical College, Manipal, India. PMID 9771390

Cancer Lett 1998 Jun 19;128(2):155-60 Inhibition by an extract of Ocimum sanctum of DNA-binding activity of 7,12-dimethylbenz[a]anthracene in rat hepatocytes in vitro. Prashar R, Kumar A, Hewer A, Cole KJ, Davis W, Phillips DH Radiation and Cancer Biology Laboratory, Department of Zoology, University of Rajasthan, Jaipur, India. PMID 9683276

Cancer Res 1998 Feb 15;58(4):717-23 Novel triterpenoids suppress inducible nitric oxide synthase (iNOS) and inducible cyclooxygenase (COX-2) in mouse macrophages. Suh N, Honda T, Finlay HJ, Barchowsky A, Williams C, Benoit NE, Xie QW, Nathan C, Gribble GW, Sporn MB Department of Pharmacology and Norris Cotton Cancer Center, Dartmouth Medical School, Hanover, New Hampshire 03755, USA. PMID 9485026

Mutat Res 1998 Feb 2;397(2):303-12 Enhancement of bone marrow radioprotection and reduction of WR-2721 toxicity by Ocimum sanctum. Ganasoundari A, Devi PU, Rao BS Department of Radiobiology, Kasturba Medical College, Manipal, Karnataka, India. PMID 9541656

Free Radic Res 1997 Aug;27(2):221-8 Evaluation of antioxidant effectiveness of a few herbal plants. Maulik G, Maulik N, Bhandari V, Kagan VE, Pakrashi S, Das DK University of Connecticut School of Medicine, Farmington, CT 06030-1110, USA. PMID 9350426

Indian J Exp Biol 1997 Apr;35(4):380-3 Evaluation of antiinflammatory activity of fatty acids of Ocimum sanctum fixed oil. Singh S, Majumdar DK College of Pharmacy (University of Delhi) Pushp Vihar, New Delhi, India. PMID 9315239

Mutat Res 1997 Feb 3;373(2):271-6 Protection against radiation-induced chromosome damage in mouse bone marrow by Ocimum sanctum. Ganasoundari A, Devi PU, Rao MN Department of Radiobiology, Dr. T.M.A. Pai Research Centre, Kasturba Medical College, Manipal, India. PMID 9042410

Indian J Exp Biol 1996 Dec;34(12):1212-5 Chemical and pharmacological studies on fixed oil of Ocimum sanctum. Singh S, Majumdar DK, Yadav MR College of Pharmacy (University of Delhi) Pushp Vihar, India. PMID 9246913

J Ethnopharmacol 1996 Oct;54(1):19-26 Evaluation of anti-inflammatory potential of fixed oil of Ocimum sanctum (Holybasil) and its possible mechanism of action. Singh S, Majumdar DK, Rehan HM College of Pharmacy (University of Delhi), New Delhi, India. PMID 8941864

Nutr Cancer 1996;25(2):205-17 Modulatory influence of alcoholic extract of Ocimum leaves on carcinogen-metabolizing enzyme activities and reduced glutathione levels in mouse. Banerjee S, Prashar R, Kumar A, Rao AR Cancer Biology Laboratory, School of Life Sciences, Jawaharlal Nehru University, New Delhi, India. PMID 8710690

Indian J Exp Biol 1995 Mar;33(3):205-8 Radioprotective effect of leaf extract of Indian medicinal plant Ocimum sanctum. Devi PU, Ganasoundari A Department of Radiobiology, Dr. T.M.A. Pai Research Centre, Kasturba Medical College, Manipal, India. PMID 7601491

Anticancer Drugs 1994 Oct;5(5):567-72 Chemopreventive action by an extract from Ocimum sanctum on mouse skin papillomagenesis and its enhancement of skin glutathione S-transferase activity and acid soluble sulfydryl level. Prashar R, Kumar A, Banerjee S, Rao AR Department of Zoology, University of Rajasthan, India. PMID 7858289

Indian J Physiol Pharmacol 1993 Jan;37(1):91-2 Ocimum sanctum Linn—a study on gastric ulceration and gastric secretion in rats. Mandal S, Das DN, De K, Ray K, Roy G, Chaudhuri SB, Sahana CC, Chowdhuri MK Department of Pharmacology, Burdwan Medical College, West Bengal. PMID 8449557

Food Chem Toxicol 1992 Nov;30(11):953-6 Anticarcinogenic effects of some Indian plant products. Aruna K, Sivaramakrishnan VM Isotope Division, Cancer Institute, Adyar, Madras, India. PMID 1473788

FEBS Lett 1992 Mar 16;299(3):213-7 Characterization of ursolic acid as a lipoxygenase and cyclooxygenase inhibitor using macrophages, platelets and differentiated HL60 leukemic cells. Najid A, Simon A, Cook J, Chable-Rabinovitch H, Delage C, Chulia AJ, Rigaud M CJF INSERM 88-03, Faculte de Medecine, Universite de Limoges, France.

J Ethnopharmacol 1987 Nov;21(2):153-63 Ocimum sanctum: an experimental study evaluating its anti-inflammatory, analgesic and antipyretic activity in animals. Godhwani S, Godhwani JL, Vyas DS Department of Pharmacology and Experimental Therapeutics, Sardar Patel Medical College, Rajasthan, India. PMID 3501819

* For resources on ursolic acid, see rosemary.

Chapter Ten: Turmeric

Clin Immunol 1999 Nov;93(2):152-61 Curcumin causes the growth arrest and apoptosis of B cell lymphoma by downregulation of egr-1, c-myc, bcl-XL, NF-kappa B, and p53. Han SS, Chung ST, Robertson DA, Ranjan D, Bondada S Department of Microbiology and Immunology, Department of General Surgery, Lexington, Kentucky 40536, USA. PMID 10527691

Oncogene 1999 Oct 28;18(44):6013-20 Inhibition of cyclo-oxygenase 2 expression in colon cells by the chemopreventive agent curcumin involves inhibition of NF-kappaB activation via the NIK/IKK signalling complex. Plummer SM, Holloway KA, Manson MM, Munks RJ, Kaptein A, Farrow S, Howells L MRC Toxicology Unit, University of Leicester, Leicester, LE1 9HN, UK. PMID 10557090

Biochem Pharmacol 1999 Oct 1;58(7):1167-72 Inhibitory effect of curcumin, a food spice from turmeric, on platelet-activating factor- and arachidonic acid-mediated platelet aggregation through inhibition of thromboxane formation and Ca2+ signaling. Shah BH, Nawaz Z, Pertani SA, Roomi A, Mahmood H, Saeed SA, Gilani AH Department of Physiology and Pharmacology, The Aga Khan University, Karachi, Pakistan. bukhtiar.shah@aku.edu PMID 10484074

Food Chem Toxicol 1999 Sep-Oct;37(9-10):985-92 Phenolics: blocking agents for heterocyclic amine-induced carcinogenesis. Hirose M, Takahashi S, Ogawa K, Futakuchi M, Shirai T First Department of Pathology, Nagoya City University, Medical School, Nagoya, Japan. PMID 10541455

Wound Repair Regen 1999 Sep-Oct;7(5):362-74 Curcumin enhances wound healing in streptozotocin induced diabetic rats and genetically diabetic mice. Sidhu GS, Mani H, Gaddipati JP, Singh AK, Seth P, Banaudha KK, Patnaik GK, Maheshwari RK Center for Combat and Life Sustainment Research, Uniformed Services University of Health Sciences, Bethesda, MD 20814, USA. rmaheshwari@usuhs.mil PMID 10564565

Toxicol Lett 1999 Sep 20;109(1-2):87-95 The effect of curcumin on glutathione-linked enzymes in K562 human leukemia cells. Singhal SS, Awasthi S, Pandya U, Piper JT, Saini MK, Cheng JZ, Awasthi YC Department of Internal Medicine, The University of Texas Medical Branch, Galveston 77555, USA. PMID 10514034

Indian J Gastroenterol 1999 Jul-Sep;18(3):118-21 Epidemiology of digestive tract cancers in India. V. Large and small bowel. Mohandas KM, Desai DC Division of Digestive Diseases and Nutrition, Tata Memorial Hospital, Mumbai. PMID 10407566

FEBS Lett 1999 Aug 6;456(2):311-4 Curcumin mediated apoptosis in AK-5 tumor cells involves the production of reactive oxygen intermediates. Bhaumik S, Anjum R, Rangaraj N, Pardhasaradhi BV, Khar A Centre for Cellular and Molecular Biology, Hyderabad, India. PMID 10456330

Chem Biol Interact 1999 Jul 1;121(2):161-75 Pro-oxidant, anti-oxidant and cleavage activities on DNA of curcumin and its derivatives demethoxycurcumin and bisdemethoxycurcumin. Ahsan H, Parveen N, Khan NU, Hadi SM Department of Biochemistry, Faculty of Life Sciences, Aligarh Muslim University, India. PMID 10418962

Cancer Lett 1999 Jul 1;141(1-2):159-65 Anti-metastatic activity of curcumin and catechin. Menon LG, Kuttan R, Kuttan G Amala Cancer Research Centre, Trichur, India. PMID 10454257

Clin Cancer Res 1999 Jul;5(7):1884-91 Curcumin inhibits tyrosine kinase activity of p185neu and also depletes p185neu. Hong RL, Spohn WH, Hung MC Department of Oncology, National Taiwan University Hospital, Taipei. PMID 10430096

Carcinogenesis 1999 Jun;20(6):1011-8 Chemoprevention by curcumin during the promotion stage of tumorigenesis of mammary gland in rats irradiated with gamma-rays. Inano H, Onoda M, Inafuku N, Kubota M, Kamada Y, Osawa T, Kobayashi H, Wakabayashi K First Research Group, National Institute of Radiological Sciences, 9-1 Anagawa-4-chome, Inage-ku, Chiba-shi 263-8555, Japan. PMID 10357781

Carcinogenesis 1999 Apr;20(4):641-4 Chemoprevention of colonic aberrant crypt foci by an inducible nitric oxide synthase-selective inhibitor. Rao CV, Kawamori T, Hamid R, Reddy BS Chemoprevention Program, American Health Foundation, Valhalla, NY 10595, USA. anshacvr@ix.netcom.com PMID 10223193

Carcinogenesis 1999 Mar;20(3):445-51 Curcumin inhibits cyclooxygenase-2 transcription in bile acid- and phorbol ester-treated human gastrointestinal epithelial cells. Zhang F, Altorki NK, Mestre JR, Subbaramaiah K, Dannenberg AJ Department of Cardiothoracic Surgery, New York Presbyterian Hospital and Weill Medical College of Cornell University, NY 10021, USA. PMID 10190560

Pharmacol Res 1999 Mar;39(3):175-9 Dietary curcumin with cisplatin administration modulates tumour marker indices in experimental fibrosarcoma. Navis I, Sriganth P, Premalatha B Departmant of Madical Biochemistry, University of Madras, Taramani Campus, Chennai, 600 113, India. PMID 10094841

FEBS Lett 1999 Feb 19;445(1):165-8 Antitumor activity of curcumin is mediated through the induction of apoptosis in AK-5 tumor cells. Khar A, Ali AM, Pardhasaradhi BV, Begum Z, Anjum R Centre for Cellular and Molecular Biology, Hyderabad, India. khar@ccmb.ap.nic.in PMID 10069393

Cancer Res 1999 Feb 1;59(3):597-601 Chemopreventive effect of curcumin, a naturally occurring anti-inflammatory agent, during the promotion/progression stages of colon cancer. Kawamori T, Lubet R, Steele VE, Kelloff GJ, Kaskey RB, Rao CV, Reddy BS Division of Nutritional Carcinogenesis, American Health Foundation, Valhalla, New York 10595, USA. PMID 9973206

Teratog Carcinog Mutagen 1999;19(1):9-18 Potentiation by turmeric and curcumin of gamma-radiation-induced chromosome aberrations in Chinese hamster ovary cells. Araujo MC, Dias FL, Takahashi CS Department of Genetics, Federal University of Pernambuco, Brazil. mcaraujo@spider.usp.br PMID 10321406

Indian J Med Res 1998 Nov;108:167-81 Bioactive phytochemicals with emphasis on dietary practices. Krishnaswamy K, Raghuramulu N National Institute of Nutrition (ICMR), Hyderabad. PMID 9863273

J Invest Dermatol 1998 Oct;111(4):656-61 Curcumin induces a p53-dependent apoptosis in human basal cell carcinoma cells. Jee SH, Shen SC, Tseng CR, Chiu HC, Kuo ML Department of Dermatology, College of Medicine, National Taiwan University, Taipei. PMID 9764849

Cell Stress Chaperones 1998 Sep;3(3):152-60 Stimulation of the stress-induced expression of stress proteins by curcumin in cultured cells and in rat tissues in vivo. Kato K, Ito H, Kamei K, Iwamoto I Department of Biochemistry, Institute for Developmental Research, Aichi Human Service Center, Kasugai, Japan. PMID 9764755

Carcinogenesis 1998 Aug;19(8):1357-60 Mechanism of inhibition of benzo[a]pyrene-induced forestomach cancer in mice by dietary curcumin. Singh SV, Hu X, Srivastava SK, Singh M, Xia H, Orchard JL, Zaren HA Cancer Research Laboratory, Mercy Cancer Institute, Pittsburgh, PA 15219, USA. PMID 9744529

Cancer Lett 1998 Jul 3;129(1):111-6 Inhibitory effect of curcuminoids on MCF-7 cell proliferation and structure-activity relationships. Simon A, Allais DP, Duroux JL, Basly JP, Durand-Fontanier S, Delage C Laboratoire de Chimie Physique et Minerale, Faculte de Pharmacie, Limoges, France. PMID 9714342

Biochem Pharmacol 1998 Jun 15;55(12):1955-62 In vivo inhibition of nitric oxide synthase gene expression by curcumin, a cancer preventive natural product with anti-inflammatory properties. Chan MM, Huang HI, Fenton MR, Fong D Department of Biomedical Sciences, Pennsylvania College of Podiatric Medicine, Philadelphia 19107, USA. chan@biology.rutgers.edu PMID 9714315

Jpn J Cancer Res 1998 Apr;89(4):361-70 Inhibitory effects of curcumin and tetrahydrocurcuminoids on the tumor promoter-induced reactive oxygen species generation in leukocytes in vitro and in vivo. Nakamura Y, Ohto Y, Murakami A, Osawa T, Ohigashi H Division of Applied Life Sciences, Graduate School of Agriculture, Kyoto University. PMID 9617340

Biochem Pharmacol 1998 Apr 15;55(8):1333-7 Nonselective inhibition of proliferation of transformed and nontransformed cells by the anticancer agent curcumin (diferuloylmethane). Gautam SC, Xu YX, Pindolia KR, Janakiraman N, Chapman RA Department of Medicine, Henry Ford Hospital, Detroit, MI 48202, USA. PMID 9719490

Int J Biochem Cell Biol 1998 Apr;30(4):445-56 Mechanisms of anticarcinogenic properties of curcumin: the effect of curcumin on glutathione linked detoxification enzymes in rat liver. Piper JT, Singhal SS, Salameh MS, Torman RT, Awasthi YC, Awasthi S Department of Internal Medicine, University of Texas Medical Branch, Galveston 77555-1067, USA. PMID 9675878

Wound Repair Regen 1998 Mar-Apr;6(2):167-77 Enhancement of wound healing by curcumin in animals. Sidhu GS, Singh AK, Thaloor D, Banaudha KK, Patnaik GK, Srimal RC, Maheshwari RK Center for Combat Casualty and Life Sustainment Research, Department of Pathology, Uniformed Services University of the Health Sciences, Bethesda, MD, USA. PMID 9776860

Carcinogenesis 1998 Mar;19(3):419-24 Quantitation of chemopreventive synergism between (-)-epigallocatechin-3-gallate and curcumin in normal, premalignant and malignant human oral epithelial cells. Khafif A, Schantz SP, Chou TC, Edelstein D, Sacks PG Department of Surgery, Head and Neck Surgery, Memorial Sloan-Kettering Cancer Center, New York, NY 10021, USA. PMID 9525275

Cancer Lett 1998 Jan 16;123(1):35-40 Chemopreventive efficacy of curcumin-free aqueous turmeric extract in 7,12-dimethylbenz[a]anthracene-induced rat mammary tumorigenesis. Deshpande SS, Ingle AD, Maru GB Carcinogenesis Division, Cancer Research Institute, Tata Memorial Centre, Parel, Mumbai, India. PMID 9461015

Free Radic Biol Med 1998 Jan 1;24(1):49-54 Effect of turmeric, turmerin and curcumin on H2O2-induced renal epithelial (LLC-PK1) cell injury. Cohly HH, Taylor A, Angel MF, Salahudeen AK Department of Surgery (Plastic), University of Mississippi Medical Center, Jackson 39216, USA. cohly@fiona.umsmed.edu PMID 9436613

Nutr Cancer 1998;30(2):163-6 Retardation of experimental tumorigenesis and reduction in DNA adducts by turmeric and curcumin. Krishnaswamy K, Goud VK, Sesikeran B, Mukundan MA, Krishna TP National Institute of Nutrition, Indian Council of Medical Research, Jamai-osmania, Hyderabad, India. PMID 9589436

FEBS Lett 1997 Nov 10;417(2):196-8 Inhibitory effect on curcumin on mammalian phospholipase D activity. Yamamoto H, Hanada K, Kawasaki K, Nishijima M Department of Biochemistry and Cell Biology, National Institute of Infectious Diseases, Toyama, Tokyo, Japan. PMID 9395294

Cancer Lett 1997 Sep 16;118(1):79-85 Inhibitory effects of curcumin-free aqueous turmeric extract on benzo[a]pyrene-induced forestomach papillomas in mice. Deshpande SS, Ingle AD, Maru GB nCarcinogenesis Division, Cancer Research Institute, Tata Memorial Centre, Parel, India. PMID 9310263

Anticancer Drugs 1997 Jun;8(5):470-81 Antiproliferative effect of curcumin (diferuloylmethane) against human breast tumor cell lines. Mehta K, Pantazis P, McQueen T, Aggarwal BB Department of Bioimmunotherapy, The University of Texas MD Anderson Cancer Center, Houston 77030, USA. PMID 9215611

Cancer Lett 1997 May 19;115(2):129-33 Protective effect of food additives on aflatoxin-induced mutagenicity and hepatocarcinogenicity. Soni KB, Lahiri M, Chackradeo P, Bhide SV, Kuttan R Amala Cancer Research Centre, Kerala State, India. PMID 9149115

Biochem Biophys Res Commun 1997 Apr 28;233(3):692-6 Curcumin and genistein, plant natural products, show synergistic inhibitory effects on the growth of human breast cancer MCF-7 cells induced by estrogenic pesticides. Verma SP, Salamone E, Goldin B Department of Community Health. Tufts University School of Medicine, Boston, Massachusetts 02111, USA. PMID 9168916

Mol Cell Biochem 1997 Apr;169(1-2):125-34 Presence of an acidic glycoprotein in the serum of arthritic rats: modulation by capsaicin and curcumin. Joe B, Rao UJ, Lokesh BR Department of Biochemistry and Nutrition, Central Food Technological Research Institute, India. PMID 9089639

Carcinogenesis 1997 Jan;18(1):83-8 Inhibitory effects of topical application of low doses of curcumin on 12-O-tetradecanoylphorbol-13-acetate-induced tumor promotion and oxidized DNA bases in mouse epidermis. Huang MT, Ma W, Yen P, Xie JG, Han J, Frenkel K, Grunberger D, Conney AH Department of Chemical Biology, College of Pharmacy, Rutgers, The State University of New Jersey, Piscataway 08855-0789, USA. PMID 9054592

J Pharm Pharmacol 1997 Jan;49(1):105-7 Nitric oxide scavenging by curcuminoids. Sreejayan, Rao MN Department of Pharmaceutical Chemistry, College of Pharmaceutical Sciences, Manipal, India. PMID 9120760

J Cell Biochem Suppl 1997;27:26-34 Inhibitory effects of curcumin on tumorigenesis in mice. Huang MT, Newmark HL, Frenkel K Department of Chemical Biology, College of Pharmacy, Rutgers-State University of New Jersey, Piscataway, NJ 08854-8020, USA. PMID 9591190

J Cell Biochem Suppl 1997;28-29:39-48 Suppression of protein kinase C and nuclear oncogene expression as possible molecular mechanisms of cancer chemoprevention by apigenin and curcumin. Lin JK, Chen YC, Huang YT, Lin-Shiau SY College of Medicine, National Taiwan University, Taipei, Taiwan. PMID 9589348

Neurobiol Dis 1997;4(3-4):137-69 Zinc metabolism in the brain: relevance to human neurodegenerative disorders. Cuajungco MP, Lees GJ Department of Psychiatry and Behavioural Science, University of Auckland School of Medicine, New Zealand. PMID 9361293

Proc Annu Meet Am Assoc Cancer Res; 38:A2850 1997 Induction of apoptosis through modulation of HSP70, calcium ion and cellular p53 protein by curcumin in colorectal carcinoma cells (Meeting abstract). Lin JK - Lin JK; Chen YC; Kuo TC; Lin-Shiau SY Institute of Biochemistry, College of Medicine, National Taiwan University, Taipei, Taiwan, ROC PMID 98639850

Cancer Lett 1996 Jun 5;103(2):137-41 Inhibition of 7,12 dimethylbenz [a]anthracene (DMBA)-induced mammary tumorigenesis and DMBA-DNA adduct formation by curcumin. Singletary K, MacDonald C, Wallig M, Fisher C Department of Food Science and Human Nutrition, University of Illinois, Urbana 61801, USA. PMID 8635149

Carcinogenesis 1996 Jun;17(6):1305-11 Effects of the phytochemicals, curcumin and quercetin, upon azoxymethane-induced colon cancer and 7,12-dimethylbenz[a]anthracene-induced mammary cancer in rats. Pereira MA, Grubbs CJ, Barnes LH, Li H, Olson GR, Eto I, Juliana M, Whitaker LM, Kelloff GJ, Steele VE, Lubet RA Environmental Health Research and Testing, Inc., Lexington, KY, USA.

Life Sci 1996;59(7):545-57 Amyloidogenic processing of Alzheimer's amyloid precursor protein in vitro and its modulation by metal ions and tacrine. Chong YH, Suh YH Department of Microbiology, College of Medicine, Ewha Womans University, Seoul, Korea. PMID 8761343

Proc Annu Meet Am Assoc Cancer Res; 37:A4103 1996 Curcumin inhibits prostaglandin synthesis and cyclooxygenase-2 expression in oral epithelial cells (Meeting abstract). Kelley DJ - Memorial Sloan-Kettering Cancer Center, New York, NY 10021 Kelley DJ; Sacks PG; Ramonetti JT; Schantz SP; Dannenberg AJ PMID 97634103

Carcinogenesis 1995 Oct;16(10):2493-7 Effects of curcumin, demethoxycurcumin, bisdemethoxycurcumin and tetrahydrocurcumin on 12-O-tetradecanoylphorbol-13-acetate-induced tumor promotion. Huang MT, Ma W, Lu YP, Chang RL, Fisher C, Manchand PS, Newmark HL, Conney AH Department of Chemical Biology and Pharmacognosy, College of Pharmacy, Rutgers State University of New Jersey, Piscataway 08855-0789, USA. PMID 7586157

Cancer Lett 1995 Sep 4;96(1):23-9 Effects of three dietary phytochemicals from tea, rosemary and turmeric on inflammation-induced nitrite production. Chan MM, Ho CT, Huang HI Department of Biological Sciences, Rutgers, State University of New Jersey, Piscataway 08855-1059, USA. PMID 7553604

Cancer Lett 1995 Jul 20;94(1):79-83 Anti-tumour and antioxidant activity of natural curcuminoids. Ruby AJ, Kuttan G, Babu KD, Rajasekharan KN, Kuttan R Amala Cancer Research Centre, Kerala, India. PMID 7621448

J Ethnopharmacol 1995 Jul 7;47(2):59-67 The anti-oxidant activity of turmeric (Curcuma longa). Selvam R, Subramanian L, Gayathri R, Angayarkanni N Department of Medical Biochemistry, Dr. A.L. Mudaliar Post Graduate Institute of Basic Medical Sciences, University of Madras, Taramani, India. PMID 7500637

Prostaglandins Leukot Essent Fatty Acids 1995 Apr;52(4):223-7 Curcumin, a major component of food spice turmeric (Curcuma longa) inhibits aggregation and alters eicosanoid metabolism in human blood platelets. Srivastava KC, Bordia A, Verma SK Department of Environmental Medicine, Odense University, Denmark. PMID 7784468

Biochem Biophys Res Commun 1995 Jan 17;206(2):533-40 Curcumin, an anti-tumour promoter and anti-inflammatory agent, inhibits induction of nitric oxide synthase in activated macrophages. Brouet I, Ohshima H Unit of Endogenous Cancer Risk Factors, International Agency for Research on Cancer, Lyon, France. PMID 7530002

Cancer Res 1995 Jan 15;55(2):259-66 Chemoprevention of colon carcinogenesis by dietary curcumin, a naturally occurring plant phenolic compound. Rao CV, Rivenson A, Simi B, Reddy BS Division of Nutritional Carcinogenesis, American Health Foundation, Valhalla, New York 10595. PMID 7812955

Mutat Res 1994 Dec 1;311(2):249-55 Diminution of singlet oxygen-induced DNA damage by curcumin and related antioxidants. Subramanian M, Sreejayan, Rao MN, Devasagayam TP, Singh BB Radiation Biology and Biochemistry Division, Bhabha Atomic Research Centre, Bombay, India. PMID 7526190

J Ethnopharmacol 1994 Dec;44(3):211-7 Adjuvant chemoprevention of experimental cancer: catechin and dietary turmeric in forestomach and oral cancer models. Azuine MA, Bhide SV Division of Pharmaceutical Microbiology and Biotechnology, National Institute for Pharmaceutical Research and Development, Abuja, Nigeria. PMID 7898128

Cancer Res 1994 Nov 15;54(22):5841-7 Inhibitory effects of dietary curcumin on forestomach, duodenal, and colon carcinogenesis in mice. Huang MT, Lou YR, Ma W, Newmark HL, Reuhl KR, Conney AH Department of Chemical Biology and Pharmacognosy, College of Pharmacy, Rutgers, State University of New Jersey, Piscataway 08855-0789. PMID 7954412

Biochim Biophys Acta 1994 Nov 10;1224(2):255-63 Role of capsaicin, curcumin and dietary n-3 fatty acids in lowering the generation of reactive oxygen species in rat peritoneal macrophages. Joe B, Lokesh BR Department of Biochemistry and Nutrition, Central Food Technological Research Institute, Mysore, India. PMID 7981240

Mol Cell Biochem 1994 Aug 17;137(1):1-8 Studies on the inhibitory effects of curcumin and eugenol on the formation of reactive oxygen species and the oxidation of ferrous iron. Reddy AC, Lokesh BR Department of Biochemistry and Nutrition, Central Food Technological Research Institute, Mysore, India. PMID 7845373

Breast Cancer Res Treat 1994;30(3):233-42 Chemoprevention of mammary tumor virus-induced and chemical carcinogen-induced rodent mammary tumors by natural plant products. Bhide SV, Azuine MA, Lahiri M, Telang NT Carcinogenesis Division, Cancer Research Institute, Bombay, India. PMID 7526904

Ann Nutr Metab 1994;38(6):349-58 Studies on anti-inflammatory activity of spice principles and dietary n-3 polyunsaturated fatty acids on carrageenan-induced inflammation in rats. Reddy AC, Lokesh BR Department of Biochemistry and Nutrition, Central Food Technological Research Institute, Mysore, India. PMID 7702364

Carcinogenesis 1993 Nov;14(11):2219-25 Inhibition by dietary curcumin of azoxymethane-induced ornithine decarboxylase, tyrosine protein kinase, arachidonic acid metabolism and aberrant crypt foci formation in the rat colon. Rao CV, Simi B, Reddy BS Division of Nutritional Carcinogenesis, American Health Foundation, Valhalla, NY 10595. PMID 8242846

Plant Foods Hum Nutr 1993 Jul;44(1):87-92 Effect of turmeric on xenobiotic metabolising enzymes. Goud VK, Polasa K, Krishnaswamy K Food and Drug Toxicology Research Centre, National Institute of Nutrition, Jamai-Osmania, Hyderabad, India. PMID 8332589

Arzneimittelforschung 1992 Jul;42(7):962-4 Induction of glutathione S-transferase activity by curcumin in mice. Susan M, Rao MN Department of Pharmaceutical Chemistry, College of Pharmaceutical Sciences, Manipal, India. PMID 1418063

J Am Coll Nutr 1992 Apr;11(2):192-8 Curcumin as an inhibitor of cancer. Nagabhushan M, Bhide SV Carcinogenesis Division, Cancer Research Institute, Bombay, India. PMID 1578097

Mutagenesis 1992 Mar;7(2):107-9 Effect of turmeric on urinary mutagens in smokers. Polasa K, Raghuram TC, Krishna TP, Krishnaswamy K National Institute of Nutrition, Jamai-osmania, Hyderabad, India. PMID 1579064

Arch Biochem Biophys 1992 Feb 1;292(2):617-23 Turmerin: a water soluble antioxidant peptide from turmeric. Srinivas L, Shalini VK, Shylaja M Department of Nutrition and Food Safety, Central Food Technological Research Institute, Karnataka State, India. PMID 1731625

Nutr Cancer 1992;17(1):77-83 Chemopreventive effect of turmeric against stomach and skin tumors induced by chemical carcinogens in Swiss mice. Azuine MA, Bhide SV Carcinogenesis Division, Tata Memorial Centre, Parel, Bombay, India. PMID 1574446

J Cancer Res Clin Oncol 1992;118(6):447-52 Protective role of aqueous turmeric extract against mutagenicity of direct-acting carcinogens as well as benzo [alpha] pyrene-induced genotoxicity and carcinogenicity. Azuine MA, Kayal JJ, Bhide SV Carcinogenesis Division, Tata Memorial Centre, Parel, Bombay, India. PMID 1618892

Food Chem Toxicol 1991 Oct;29(10):699-706 Turmeric (Curcuma longa)-induced reduction in urinary mutagens. Polasa K, Sesikaran B, Krishna TP, Krishnaswamy K National Institute of Nutrition, Jamai-Osmania, Hyderabad, A.P., India. PMID 1660015

Cancer Res 1991 Feb 1;51(3):813-9 Inhibitory effects of curcumin on in vitro lipoxygenase and cyclooxygenase activities in mouse epidermis. Huang MT, Lysz T, Ferraro T, Abidi TF, Laskin JD, Conney AH Department of Chemical Biology and Pharmacognosy, College of Pharmacy, Rutgers, State University of New Jersey, Piscataway, New Jersey 0885-0789. PMID 1899046

Adv Enzyme Regul 1991;31:385-96 Inhibitory effect of curcumin and some related dietary compounds on tumor promotion and arachidonic acid metabolism in mouse skin. Conney AH, Lysz T, Ferraro T, Abidi TF, Manchand PS, Laskin JD, Huang MT Department of Chemical Biology and Pharmacognosy, College of Pharmacy, Rutgers, State University of New Jersey, Piscataway 08855-0789. PMID 1908616

Free Radic Biol Med 1991;11(3):277-83 DNA damage by smoke: protection by turmeric and other inhibitors of ROS. Srinivas L, Shalini VK Department of Nutrition and Food Safety, Central Food Technological Research Institute, Mysore, India. PMID 1937145

Indian J Exp Biol 1990 Nov;28(11):1008-11 Plant products as protective agents against cancer. Aruna K, Sivaramakrishnan VM Isotope Division, Cancer Institute, Madras, India. PMID 2283166

J Ethnopharmacol 1990 Apr;29(1):25-34 Evaluation of turmeric (Curcuma longa) for gastric and duodenal antiulcer activity in rats. Rafatullah S, Tariq M, Al-Yahya MA, Mossa JS, Ageel AM Medicinal, Aromatic and Poisonous Plants Research Center, College of Pharmacy, King Saud University, Riyadh, Saudi Arabia. PMID 2345457

Prostaglandins Leukot Essent Fatty Acids 1989 Jul;37(1):57-64 Extracts from two frequently consumed spices—cumin (Cuminum cyminum) and turmeric (Curcuma longa)—inhibit platelet aggregation and alter eicosanoid biosynthesis in human blood platelets. Srivastava KC Department of Environmental Medicine, Odense University, Denmark. PMID 2503839

Cancer Res 1988 Nov 1;48(21):5941-6 Inhibitory effect of curcumin, chlorogenic acid, caffeic acid, and ferulic acid on tumor promotion in mouse skin by 12-O-tetradecanoylphorbol-13-acetate. Huang MT, Smart RC, Wong CQ, Conney AH Department of Chemical Biology and Pharmacognosy, College of Pharmacy, Rutgers, State University of New Jersey, Piscataway 08855-0789. PMID 3139287

Tumori 1987 Feb 28;73(1):29-31 Turmeric and curcumin as topical agents in cancer therapy. Kuttan R, Sudheeran PC, Josph CD PMID 2435036

Int J Clin Pharmacol Ther Toxicol 1986 Dec;24(12):651-4 Evaluation of anti-inflammatory property of curcumin (diferuloyl methane) in patients with postoperative inflammation. Satoskar RR, Shah SJ, Shenoy SG PMID 3546166

Cancer Lett 1985 Nov;29(2):197-202 Potential anticancer activity of turmeric (Curcuma longa). Kuttan R, Bhanumathy P, Nirmala K, George MC PMID 4075289

Agents Actions 1982 Oct;12(4):508-15 Anti-inflammatory and irritant activities of curcumin analogues in rats. Mukhopadhyay A, Basu N, Ghatak N, Gujral PK PMID 7180736

Chapter Eleven: Baikal Skullcap*

Biochem Biophys Res Commun 1999 Dec 20;266(2):392-9 Lipoxygenase inhibition induced apoptosis, morphological changes, and carbonic anhydrase expression in human pancreatic cancer cells. Ding XZ, Kuszynski CA, El-Metwally TH, Adrian TE Department of Biomedical Sciences, Creighton University School of Medicine, Omaha, Nebraska, 68178, USA PMID 10600514

Biochim Biophys Acta 1999 Nov 16;1472(3):643-50 Free radical scavenging and antioxidant activities of flavonoids extracted from the radix of scutellaria baicalensis georgi. Gao Z, Huang K, Yang X, Xu H Department of Chemistry, Huazhong University of Science and Technology, Wuhan, PR China. PMID 10564778

J Mol Cell Cardiol 1999 Oct;31(10):1885-95 Extract from Scutellaria baicalensis Georgi attenuates oxidant stress in cardiomyocytes. Shao ZH, Li CQ, Vanden Hoek TL, Becker LB, Schumacker PT, Wu JA, Attele AS, Yuan CS Pritzker School of Medicine, University of Chicago, Chicago, Illinois 60637, USA. PMID 10525426

Pharmacol Toxicol 1999 Jun;84(6):288-91 Inhibitory effects of baicalein and wogonin on lipopolysaccharide-induced nitric oxide production in macrophages. Wakabayashi I Department of Hygiene and Preventive Medicine, School of Medicine, Yamagata University, Japan. PMID 10401731

Prostaglandins Other Lipid Mediat 1999 May;57(2-3):119-31 Role of prostaglandin H synthase isoforms in murine ear edema induced by phorbol ester application on skin. Sanchez T, Moreno JJ Department of Physiological Sciences, School of Pharmacy, Barcelona University, Spain.

Arch Pharm Res 1999 Feb;22(1):18-24 Inhibition of cyclooxygenase/lipoxygenase from human platelets by polyhydroxylated/methoxylated flavonoids isolated from medicinal plants. You KM, Jong HG, Kim HP College of Pharmacy, Kangwon National University, Chunchon, Korea. PMID 10071954

Nutr Cancer 1999;34(2):185-91 Inhibitory effect of 12-O-tetradecanoylphorbol-13-acetate-caused tumor promotion in benzo[a]pyrene-initiated CD-1 mouse skin by baicalein. Lee MJ, Wang CJ, Tsai YY, Hwang JM, Lin WL, Tseng TH, Chu CY Institute of Biochemistry, Chung Shan Medical and Dental College Hospital, Taichung, Taiwan. PMID 10578486

Eur J Cancer Prev 1998 Dec;7(6):465-71 Induction of quinone reductase by a methanol extract of Scutellaria baicalensis and its flavonoids in murine Hepa 1c1c7 cells. Park HJ, Lee YW, Park HH, Lee YS, Kwon IB, Yu JH Department of Biological Science, Lotte Group R & D Center, Seoul, Korea. PMID 9926295

Chem Pharm Bull (Tokyo) 1998 Sep;46(9):1383-7 Protective effects of baicalein against cell damage by reactive oxygen species. Gao D, Tawa R, Masaki H, Okano Y, Sakurai H Department of Analytical and Bioinorganic Chemistry, Kyoto Pharmaceutical University, Japan. PMID 9775434

Biol Pharm Bull 1998 Aug;21(8):814-7 Inhibitory effect of Coptidis Rhizoma and Scutellariae Radix on azoxymethane-induced aberrant crypt foci formation in rat colon. Fukutake M, Yokota S, Kawamura H, Iizuka A, Amagaya S, Fukuda K, Komatsu Y Central Research Laboratories, Tsumura & Co., Ibaraki, Japan. PMID 9743248

Am J Chin Med 1998;26(3-4):311-23 Analysis of inhibitory effects of scutellariae radix and baicalein on prostaglandin E2 production in rat C6 glioma cells. Nakahata N, Kutsuwa M, Kyo R, Kubo M, Hayashi K, Ohizumi Y Department of Pharmaceutical Molecular Biology, Faculty of Pharmaceutical Sciences, Tohoku University, Sendai, Japan. PMID 9862019

Z Naturforsch [C] 1997 Nov-Dec;52(11-12):817-23 Antioxidant activity of flavones from Scutellaria baicalensis in lecithin liposomes. Gabrielska J, Oszmianski J, Zylka R, Komorowska M Department of Physics and Biophysics, Agricultural University, Norwida, Wroclaw. PMID 9463939

Brain Res 1996 Aug 19;730(1-2):40-6 Involvement of the 12-lipoxygenase pathway of arachidonic acid metabolism in homosynaptic long-term depression of the rat hippocampus. Normandin M, Gagne J, Bernard J, Elie R, Miceli D, Baudry M, Massicotte G Centre de Recherche Fernand-Seguin, Montreal, Quebec, Canada. PMID 8883886

Am J Chin Med 1996;24(1):31-6 The anti-inflammatory activity of Scutellaria rivularis extracts and its active components, baicalin, baicalein and wogonin. Lin CC, Shieh DE Graduate Institute of Natural Products, Kaohsiung Medical College, Taiwan. PMID 8739179

Res Commun Mol Pathol Pharmacol 1995 Oct;90(1):103-14 Protection by baicalein against ascorbic acid-induced lipid peroxidation of rat liver microsomes. Gao D, Sakurai K, Chen J, Ogiso T Shenyang College of Pharmacy, P.R. China. PMID 8581335

Planta Med 1995 Apr;61(2):150-3 Pharmacological effects of methanolic extract from the root of Scutellaria baicalensis and its flavonoids on human gingival fibroblast. Chung CP, Park JB, Bae KH College of Dentistry, Seoul National University, Korea. PMID 7753922

Eur J Pharmacol 1994 Jan 4;251(1):91-3 Antiproliferative effect of baicalein, a flavonoid from a Chinese herb, on vascular smooth muscle cell. Huang HC, Wang HR, Hsieh LM Department of Pharmacology, College of Medicine, National Taiwan University, Taipei, ROC. PMID 8137874

Arch Biochem Biophys 1993 Oct;306(1):261-6 Free radical scavenging action of baicalein. Hamada H, Hiramatsu M, Edamatsu R, Mori A Department of Neuroscience, Okayama University Medical School, Japan. PMID 8215413

Agents Actions 1993;39 Spec No:C49-51 Anti-inflammatory properties and inhibition of leukotriene C4 biosynthesis in vitro by flavonoid baicalein from Scutellaria baicalensis georgy roots. Butenko IG, Gladtchenko SV, Galushko SV State Scientific Center of Drugs, Kharkov, Ukraine. PMID 8273583

* For references on melatonin, see ginger.

Chapter Twelve: Hu zhang

Proc Natl Sci Counc Repub China B 1999 Jul;23(3):99-106 Chemoprevention of cancer and cardiovascular disease by resveratrol. Lin JK, Tsai SH Institute of Biochemistry, College of Medicine, National Taiwan University, Taipei, R.O.C. PMID 10492890

Cancer Lett 1999 Jun 1;140(1-2):1-10 Resveratrol, an antioxidant present in red wine, induces apoptosis in human promyelocytic leukemia (HL-60) cells. Surh YJ, Hurh YJ, Kang JY, Lee E, Kong G, Lee SJ Laboratory of Biochemistry and Molecular Toxicology, College of Pharmacy, Seoul National University, South Korea. surh@plaza.snu.ac.kr PMID 10403535

J Cell Physiol 1999 Jun;179(3):297-304 Resveratrol, a natural product derived from grape, exhibits antiestrogenic activity and inhibits the growth of human breast cancer cells. Lu R, Serrero G Department of Pharmaceutical Sciences, University of Maryland School of Pharmacy, Baltimore 21201, USA. PMID 10228948

Br J Pharmacol 1999 Feb;126(3):673-80 Suppression of nitric oxide synthase and the down-regulation of the activation of NFkappaB in macrophages by resveratrol. Tsai SH, Lin-Shiau SY, Lin JK Institute of Biochemistry, College of Medicine, National Taiwan University, Taipei, ROC. PMID 10188978

Biochem Biophys Res Commun 1999 Jan 27;254(3):739-43 Resveratrol, a natural product present in wine, decreases tumour growth in a rat tumour model. Carbo N, Costelli P, Baccino FM, Lopez-Soriano FJ, Argiles JM Departament de Bioquimica i Biologia Molecular, Facultat de Biologia, Universitat de Barcelona, Barcelona, Spain. PMID 9920811

Drugs Exp Clin Res 1999;25(2-3):111-4 Nonalcoholic compounds of wine: the phytoestrogen resveratrol and moderate red wine consumption during menopause. Calabrese G Department of Human Nutrition, Universita Cattolica S. Cuore, Piacenza, Italy. PMID 10370872

Drugs Exp Clin Res 1999;25(2-3):65-77 Cancer chemopreventive activity of resveratrol. Jang M, Pezzuto JM Department of Surgical Oncology, University of Illinois at Chicago, USA. PMID 10370867

Herbs of the Bible Duke, J.A., Loveland, CO; Interweave Press 1999

Cancer Lett 1998 Dec 11;134(1):81-9 Effects of resveratrol on 12-O-tetradecanoylphorbol-13-acetate-induced oxidative events and gene expression in mouse skin. Jang M, Pezzuto JM Department of Medicinal Chemistry and Pharmacognosy, College of Pharmacy, University of Illinois at Chicago, 60612, USA. PMID 10381133

J Biol Chem 1998 Aug 21;273(34):21875-82 Resveratrol inhibits cyclooxygenase-2 transcription and activity in phorbol ester-treated human mammary epithelial cells. Subbaramaiah K, Chung WJ, Michaluart P, Telang N, Tanabe T, Inoue H, Jang M, Pezzuto JM, Dannenberg AJ Department of Medicine, Department of Surgery, at Memorial Sloan-Kettering Cancer Center, New York, New York 10021, USA. PMID 9705326

Blood 1998 Aug 1;92(3):996-1002 Chemopreventive agent resveratrol, a natural product derived from grapes, triggers CD95 signaling-dependent apoptosis in human tumor cells. Clement MV, Hirpara JL, Chawdhury SH, Pervaiz S Department of Physiology and Oncology Research Institute, NUMI, National University of Singapore, Singapore. PMID 9680369

Prostaglandins Other Lipid Mediat 1998 Jun;56(2-3):131-43 Paradoxical effects of resveratrol on the two prostaglandin H synthases. Johnson JL, Maddipati KR Division of Bioorganic Chemistry, Cayman Chemical Company, Ann Arbor, Michigan 48108, USA. PMID 9785383

Acta Biol Hung 1998;49(2-4):281-9 Identification and measurement of resveratrol and formaldehyde in parts of white and blue grape berries. Kiraly-Veghely Z, Tyihak E, Albert L, Nemeth ZI, Katay G Research Institute for Viticulture and Enology of Agricultural Ministry, Experimental Wine Cellar, Budapest, Hungary. PMID 10526971

Proc Natl Acad Sci U S A 1997 Dec 9;94(25):14138-43 Resveratrol, a polyphenolic compound found in grapes and wine, is an agonist for the estrogen receptor. Gehm BD, McAndrews JM, Chien PY, Jameson JL Division of Endocrinology, Metabolism and Molecular Medicine, Northwestern University Medical School, 303 E. Chicago Avenue, Chicago, IL 60611, USA. PMID 9391166

Science 1997 Jan 10;275(5297):218-20 Cancer chemopreventive activity of resveratrol, a natural product derived from grapes. Jang M, Cai L, Udeani GO, Slowing KV, Thomas CF, Beecher CW, Fong HH, Farnsworth NR, Kinghorn AD, Mehta RG, Moon RC, Pezzuto JM Department of Medicinal Chemistry and Pharmacognosy, College of Pharmacy, University of Illinois at Chicago, Chicago, IL 60612, USA. PMID 8985016

Science (1997;275:218-220) Resveratrol inhibits cyclooxygenase (COX), an enzyme that stimulates production of inflammatory substances that "can stimulate tumor cell growth and suppress immune surveillance"

Proc Natl Acad Sci USA 1997;94:14138-14143. Resveratrol can inhibit the binding of estradiol.

Mutat Res 1995 Jul;329(2):205-12 Emodin inhibits the mutagenicity and DNA adducts induced by 1-nitropyrene. Su HY, Cherng SH, Chen CC, Lee H Environmental Toxicological Center, Chung Shan Medical and Dental College, Taichung, Taiwan, ROC. PMID 7603502

J Nat Prod 1993 Oct;56(10):1805-10 Kinase inhibitors from Polygonum cuspidatum. Jayatilake GS, Jayasuriya H, Lee ES, Koonchanok NM, Geahlen RL, Ashendel CL, McLaughlin JL, Chang CJ Department of Medicinal Chemistry and Pharmacognosy, School of Pharmacy and Pharmacal Sciences, Purdue University, West Lafayette, Indiana 47907. PMID 8277318

Biochim Biophys Acta 1985 Apr 25;834(2):275-8 Effects of stilbenes on arachidonate metabolism in leukocytes. Kimura Y, Okuda H, Arichi S PMID 3922423

Chapter Thirteen: Rosemary

Carcinogenesis 1999 Oct;20(10):1945-52 Suppression of inducible cyclooxygenase and inducible nitric oxide synthase by apigenin and related flavonoids in mouse macrophages. Liang YC, Huang YT, Tsai SH, Lin-Shiau SY, Chen CF, Lin JK Institute of Biochemistry, College of Medicine, National Taiwan University, No. 1, Section 1, Taipei, Taiwan. PMID 10506109

J Nat Prod 1998 Oct;61(10):1212-5 Ursolic acid from Plantago major, a selective inhibitor of cyclooxygenase-2 catalyzed prostaglandin biosynthesis. Ringbom T, Segura L, Noreen Y, Perera P, Bohlin L Division of Pharmacognosy, Department of Pharmacy, Biomedical Centre, Uppsala University, Box 579, S-751 23 Uppsala, Sweden   PMID 9784154

Cancer Res 1998 Jun 1;58(11):2323-7 Antioxidants reduce cyclooxygenase-2 expression, prostaglandin production, and proliferation in colorectal cancer cells. Chinery R, Beauchamp RD, Shyr Y, Kirkland SC, Coffey RJ, Morrow JD Department of Medicine, The Vanderbilt Cancer Center, Vanderbilt University Medical Center, Nashville, Tennessee 37232, USA. PMID 9622066

Arch Toxicol Suppl 1998;20:227-36 Development of in vitro models for cellular and molecular studies in toxicology and chemoprevention. Mace K, Offord EA, Harris CC, Pfeifer AM Nestle Research Center, Lausanne, Switzerland. PMID 9442296

Cancer Lett 1997 Mar 19;114(1-2):275-81 Mechanisms involved in the chemoprotective effects of rosemary extract studied in human liver and bronchial cells. Offord EA, Mace K, Avanti O, Pfeifer AM Nestle Research Centre, Lausanne, Switzerland. elizabeth.offord-cavin@chlsnr.nestrd.ch PMID 9103309

Carcinogenesis 1995 Sep;16(9):2057-62 Rosemary components inhibit benzo[a]pyrene-induced genotoxicity in human bronchial cells. Offord EA, Mace K, Ruffieux C, Malnoe A, Pfeifer AM Nestle Research Centre, Lausanne, Switzerland. PMID 7554054

Planta Med 1995 Aug;61(4):333-6 Inhibition of lipid peroxidation and superoxide generation by diterpenoids from Rosmarinus officinalis. Haraguchi H, Saito T, Okamura N, Yagi A Faculty of Engineering, Fukuyama University, Japan. PMID 7480180

J Clin Invest 1995 Apr;95(4):1669-75 Involvement of reactive oxygen intermediates in cyclooxygenase-2 expression induced by interleukin-1, tumor necrosis factor-alpha, and lipopolysaccharide. Feng L, Xia Y, Garcia GE, Hwang D, Wilson CB Department of Immunology, Scripps Research Institute, La Jolla, California 92037, USA. PMID 7706475

J Clin Invest 1995 Apr;95(4):1669-75 Involvement of reactive oxygen intermediates in cyclooxygenase-2 expression induced by interleukin-1, tumor necrosis factor-alpha, and lipopolysaccharide. Feng L, Xia Y, Garcia GE, Hwang D, Wilson CB Department of Immunology, Scripps Research Institute, La Jolla, California 92037, USA. PMID 9622066, 7706475

Cancer Res 1994 Feb 1;54(3):701-8 Inhibition of skin tumorigenesis by rosemary and its constituents carnosol and ursolic acid. Huang MT, Ho CT, Wang ZY, Ferraro T, Lou YR, Stauber K, Ma W, Georgiadis C, Laskin JD, Conney AH Department of Chemical Biology and Pharmacognosy, College of Pharmacy, Rutgers, State University of New Jersey, Piscataway 08855-0789. PMID 8306331

Chapter Fourteen: Ginger*

J Pineal Res 1999 Aug;27(1):9-14 Regulation of prostaglandin production in carrageenan-induced pleurisy by melatonin. Cuzzocrea S, Costantino G, Mazzon E, Caputi AP Institute of Pharmacology, School of Medicine, University of Messina, Italy. salvator@imeuniv.unime.it PMID 10451019

Semin Urol Oncol 1999 May;17(2):111-8 Meditation and prostate cancer: integrating a mind/body intervention with traditional therapies. Coker KH Robert W. Woodruff Health Sciences Center, Emory University, The Emory Clinic Inc., Atlanta, GA 30022, USA. PMID 10332925

Biol Signals Recept 1999 Jan-Apr;8(1-2):49-55 New actions of melatonin on tumor metabolism and growth. Blask DE, Sauer LA, Dauchy R, Holowachuk EW, Ruhoff MS Bassett Research Institute, Mary Imogene Bassett Hospital, Cooperstown, NY 13326-1394, USA. dblask@usa.net PMID 10085462

J Natl Cancer Inst 1999 Jan 6;91(1):22-36 Inhibition of metastases by anticoagulants. Hejna M, Raderer M, Zielinski CC Department of Medicine I, University Hospital, Vienna, Austria.

Biochem. J. (1999) 344, 487–493 Melatonin: an endogenous negative modulator of 12-lipoxygenation in the rat pineal gland Hongjian ZHANG2, Mohammed AKBAR and Hee-Yong KIM1 Section of Mass Spectrometry, Laboratory of Membrane Biochemistry and Biophysics, NIAAA, NIH, 12501 Washington Avenue, Rockville, MD 20852, U.S.A.

Cancer Lett 1998 Dec 25;134(2):163-8 Induction of apoptosis in HL-60 cells by pungent vanilloids, [6]-gingerol and [6]-paradol. Lee E, Surh YJ College of Pharmacy, Seoul National University, South Korea. PMID 10025876

J Ethnopharmacol 1998 Aug;62(1):49-55 Reversal of cisplatin-induced delay in gastric emptying in rats by ginger (Zingiber officinale). Sharma SS, Gupta YK Department of Pharmacology, All India Institute of Medical Sciences, New Delhi.

Cancer Lett 1998 Jul 17;129(2):139-44 Published erratum appears in Cancer Lett 1998 Sep 25;131(2):231 Inhibitory effects of [6]-gingerol, a major pungent principle of ginger, on phorbol ester-induced inflammation, epidermal ornithine decarboxylase activity and skin tumor promotion in ICR mice. Park KK, Chun KS, Lee JM, Lee SS, Surh YJ Yonsei University College of Dentistry, Seoul, South Korea. PMID 9719454

Biol Signals Recept 1998 Jan-Feb;7(1):61-72 Melatonin involvement in immunity and cancer. Fraschini F, Demartini G, Esposti D, Scaglione F Department of Pharmacology, University of Milan, Italy. f.fraschini@unimi.it PMID 9641799

Cancer Detect Prev 1998;22(6):516-25 Screening for in vitro anti-tumor-promoting activities of edible plants from Indonesia. Murakami A, Morita H, Safitri R, Ramlan A, Koshimizu K, Ohigashi H Department of Biotechnological Science, Faculty of Biology-Oriented Science and Technology, Kinki University, Iwade-Uchita, Wakayama, Japan.

Lancet 1997 (Nov. 29): 1598-99. Murch, S., Simmons, C. and Saxena, P.

Wien Klin Wochenschr 1997 Oct 3;109(18):722-9 [Significance of melatonin in malignant diseases]. Bartsch C, Bartsch H Universitats-Frauenklinik, Tubingen, Bundesrepublik Deutschland. PMID 9441515

Cancer Res 1996 Mar 1;56(5):1023-30 Inhibition of tumor promotion in SENCAR mouse skin by ethanol extract of Zingiber officinale rhizome. Katiyar SK, Agarwal R, Mukhtar H Department of Dermatology, Skin Diseases Research Center, University Hospitals of Cleveland, Case Western Reserve University, Ohio 44106, USA. PMID 8640756

Biochem Mol Biol Int 1995 Mar;35(3):627-34 Identification of melatonin in plants and its effects on plasma melatonin levels and binding to melatonin receptors in vertebrates. Hattori A, Migitaka H, Iigo M, Itoh M, Yamamoto K, Ohtani-Kaneko R, Hara M, Suzuki T, Reiter RJ Department of Anatomy, St. Marianna University School of Medicine, Kawasaki, Japan. PMID 7773197 10451019

Pharmacology 1994 Nov;49(5):314-8 Suppressive effects of eugenol and ginger oil on arthritic rats. Sharma JN, Srivastava KC, Gan EK Department of Pharmacology, School of Medical Sciences, University of Science Malaysia, Kelantan.

Chem Pharm Bull (Tokyo) 1994 Jun;42(6):1226-30 Stomachic principles in ginger. III. An anti-ulcer principle, 6-gingesulfonic acid, and three monoacyldigalactosylglycerols, gingerglycolipids A, B, and C, from Zingiberis Rhizoma originating in Taiwan. Yoshikawa M, Yamaguchi S, Kunimi K, Matsuda H, Okuno Y, Yamahara J, Murakami N Kyoto Pharmaceutical University, Japan. PMID 8069973

Anticancer Res 1994 Mar-Apr;14(2A):501-6 Inhibitory effects of phenolics on xanthine oxidase. Chang WS, Chang YH, Lu FJ, Chiang HC School of Pharmacy, College of Medicine, National Taiwan University, Taipei, R.O.C. PMID 8017853

Teratog Carcinog Mutagen 1994;14(5):213-7 Electromagnetic fields and brain tumours: a commentary. Hughes JT Green College, University of Oxford, United Kingdom. PMID 7855741

Yakugaku Zasshi 1993 Apr;113(4):307-15 [Qualitative and quantitative analysis of bioactive principles in Zingiberis Rhizoma by means of high performance liquid chromatography and gas liquid chromatography. On the evaluation of Zingiberis Rhizoma and chemical change of constituents during Zingiberis Rhizoma processing]. Yoshikawa M, Hatakeyama S, Chatani N, Nishino Y, Yamahara J Kyoto Pharmaceutical University, Japan. PMID 8492294

Med Hypotheses 1992 Dec;39(4):342-8 Ginger (Zingiber officinale) in rheumatism and musculoskeletal disorders. Srivastava KC, Mustafa T Department of Environmental Medicine, Odense University, Denmark.

Yakugaku Zasshi 1992 Sep;112(9):645-55 [Stomachic principles in ginger. II. Pungent and anti-ulcer effects of low polar constituents isolated from ginger, the dried rhizoma of Zingiber officinale Roscoe cultivated in Taiwan. The absolute stereostructure of a new diarylheptanoid]. Yamahara J, Hatakeyama S, Taniguchi K, Kawamura M, Yoshikawa M Kyoto Pharmaceutical University, Japan. PMID 1469612

J Basic Clin Physiol Pharmacol 1992 Jan-Mar;3(1):33-40 Melatonin levels are decreased in rheumatoid arthritis. West SK, Oosthuizen JM Department of Medical Physiology and Biochemistry, Faculty of Medicine, University of Stellenbosch, Republic of South Africa. PMID 1504062

Chung Kuo Chung Yao Tsa Chih 1990 May;15(5):278-80, 317-8 [Effect of dry ginger and roasted ginger on experimental gastric ulcers in rats]. Wu H, Ye D, Bai Y, Zhao Y Nanjing College of Traditional Chinese Medicine. PMID 2275778

Med Hypotheses 1989 May;29(1):25-8 Ginger (Zingiber officinale) and rheumatic disorders.Srivastava KC, Mustafa T Department of Environmental Medicine, Odense University, Denmark.

Am J Chin Med 1989;17(1-2):51-6 Gastroprotective activity of ginger zingiber officinale rosc., in albino rats. al-Yahya MA, Rafatullah S, Mossa JS, Ageel AM, Parmar NS, Tariq M Medicinal, Aromatic and Poisonous Plants Research Center, College of Pharmacy, King Saud University, Riyadh, Saudi Arabia. PMID 2589236

J Ethnopharmacol 1988 Jul-Aug;23(2-3):299-304 The anti-ulcer effect in rats of ginger constituents. Yamahara J, Mochizuki M, Rong HQ, Matsuda H, Fujimura H Kyoto Pharmaceutical University, Japan. PMID 3193792

Nippon Yakurigaku Zasshi 1986 Oct;88(4):263-9 [Pharmacological studies on ginger. IV. Effect of (6)-shogaol on the arachidonic cascade]. Suekawa M, Yuasa K, Isono M, Sone H, Ikeya Y, Sakakibara I, Aburada M, Hosoya E PMID 3098654

Biomed Biochim Acta 1984;43(8-9):S335-46 Aqueous extracts of onion, garlic and ginger inhibit platelet aggregation and alter arachidonic acid metabolism. Srivastava KC PMID 6440548

* For references on curcumin, see turmeric.

Chapter Fifteen: Oregano

Clin Pharmacol Ther 1999 Mar;65(3):336-47 Characterization of rofecoxib as a cyclooxygenase-2 isoform inhibitor and demonstration of analgesia in the dental pain model. Ehrich EW, Dallob A, De Lepeleire I, Van Hecken A, Riendeau D, Yuan W, Porras A, Wittreich J, Seibold JR, De Schepper P, Mehlisch DR, Gertz BJ Department of Clinical Research, Merck Research Laboratories, Rahway, NJ, USA. elliot_ehrich@merck.com PMID 10096266

Proc Natl Acad Sci U S A 1999 Jan 5;96(1):272-7 Published erratum appears in Proc Natl Acad Sci U S A 1999 May 11;96(10):5890 Systemic biosynthesis of prostacyclin by cyclooxygenase (COX)-2: the human pharmacology of a selective inhibitor of COX-2. McAdam BF, Catella-Lawson F, Mardini IA, Kapoor S, Lawson JA, FitzGerald GA EUPENN Group of Investigators, Center For Experimental Therapeutics, University Of Pennsylvania, Philadelphia, PA 19104, USA. PMID 9874808

J Pharmacol Exp Ther 1998 Nov;287(2):578-82 Selective cyclooxygenase-2 inhibition by nimesulide in man. Cullen L, Kelly L, Connor SO, Fitzgerald DJ Centre for Cardiovascular Science, Royal College of Surgeons in Ireland, St. Stephens Green, Dublin 2, Ireland. PMID 9808683

Arthritis Rheum 1998 Sep;41(9):1591-602 Preliminary study of the safety and efficacy of SC-58635, a novel cyclooxygenase 2 inhibitor: efficacy and safety in two placebo-controlled trials in osteoarthritis and rheumatoid arthritis, and studies of gastrointestinal and platelet effects. Simon LS, Lanza FL, Lipsky PE, Hubbard RC, Talwalker S, Schwartz BD, Isakson PC, Geis GS Beth Israel Deaconess Medical Center, Harvard Medical School, Boston, Massachusetts 02215, USA. PMID 9751091

Acta Pharm Hung 1998 May;68(3):183-8 [Investigation of variation of the production of biological and chemical compounds of Hyssopus officinalis L]. Varga E, Hajdu Z, Veres K, Mathe I, Nemeth E, Pluhar Z, Bernath J SZOTE Gyogynoveny- es Drogismereti Intezet, Szeged. PMID: 9703705

J Nat Prod 1997 Nov;60(11):1170-3 Saniculoside N from Sanicula europaea L. Arda N, Goren N, Kuru A, Pengsuparp T, Pezzuto JM, Qiu SX, Cordell GA Department of Biology, Faculty of Science, University of Istanbul, Turkey. PMID: 9392884

Planta Med 1995 Jun;61(3):227-32 Biological and pharmacological activities and further constituents of Hyptis verticillata. Kuhnt M, Probstle A, Rimpler H, Bauer R, Heinrich M Institut fur Pharmazeutische Biologie, Albert-Ludwigs-Universitat, Freiburg, Germany. PMID: 7617764

Yao Hsueh Hsueh Pao 1993;28(4):241-5 [Antithrombotic and antiplatelet effects of rosmarinic acid, a water-soluble component isolated from radix Salviae miltiorrhizae]. Zou ZW, Xu LN, Tian JY Institute of Materia Medica, Chinese Academy of Medical Sciences, Beijing. PMID: 8213164

Yao Hsueh Hsueh Pao 1992;27(2):96-100 [Antioxidative effect of three water-soluble components isolated from Salvia miltiorrhiza in vitro]. Huang YS, Zhang JT Institute of Materia Medica, Chinese Academy of Medical Sciences, Beijing. PMID: 1414377

Int J Immunopharmacol 1991;13(7):853-7 The inhibitory effect of rosmarinic acid on complement involves the C5 convertase. Peake PW, Pussell BA, Martyn P, Timmermans V, Charlesworth JA Department of Nephrology, Prince Henry Hospital, Sydney, NSW, Australia. PMID: 1761351

Ann Pharm Fr 1990;48(2):103-8 [Rosmarinic acid, total hydroxycinnamic derivatives and antioxidant activity of Apiaceae, Borraginaceae and Lamiceae medicinals]. [Article in French] Lamaison JL, Petitjean-Freytet C, Carnat A Laboratoire de Pharmacognosie et Phytotherapie, Faculte de Pharmacie, Clermont-Ferrand. PMID: 2291599

Methods Find Exp Clin Pharmacol 1989 May;11(5):345-52 Percutaneous absorption of rosmarinic acid in the rat. Ritschel WA, Starzacher A, Sabouni A, Hussain AS, Koch HP University of Cincinnati Medical Center, Div. of Pharmaceutics and Drug Delivery Systems, OH. PMID: 2755281

289

Chapter Sixteen: Feverfew

J Ethnopharmacol 1999 Dec 15;68(1-3):251-9 Antinociceptive and anti-inflammatory effects of Tanacetum parthenium L. extract in mice and rats. Jain NK, Kulkarni SK Pharmacology Division, University Institute of Pharmaceutical Sciences, Panjab University, Chandigarh, India. [Medline record in process] PMID: 10624885

Phytochemistry 1999 Jun;51(3):417-23 The flavonoids of Tanacetum parthenium and T. vulgare and their anti-inflammatory properties. Williams CA, Harborne JB, Geiger H, Hoult JR Department of Botany, University of Reading, UK. PMID: 10382317

Planta Med 1999 Mar;65(2):126-9 Low concentrations of the feverfew component parthenolide inhibit in vitro growth of tumor lines in a cytostatic fashion. Ross JJ, Arnason JT, Birnboim HC Department of Biology, University of Ottawa, Ontario, Canada. PMID: 10193202

Cephalalgia 1998 Dec;18(10):704-8 Feverfew as a preventive treatment for migraine: a systematic review. Vogler BK, Pittler MH, Ernst E Department of Complementary Medicine, School of Postgraduate Medicine and Health Sciences, University of Exeter, UK. PMID: 9950629

Lancet 1997 Nov 29;350(9091):1598-9 Melatonin in feverfew and other medicinal plants. Murch SJ, Simmons CB, Saxena PK Publication Types: Letter PMID: 9393344

J Pharm Pharmacol 1997 May;49(5):558-61 Pharmacological activity of feverfew (Tanacetum parthenium (L.) Schultz-Bip.): assessment by inhibition of human polymorphonuclear leukocyte chemiluminescence in-vitro. Brown AM, Edwards CM, Davey MR, Power JB, Lowe KC Department of Life Science, University of Nottingham, University Park, UK. PMID: 9178194

Biochem Biophys Res Commun 1996 Sep 24;226(3):810-8 Inhibition of the expression of inducible cyclooxygenase and proinflammatory cytokines by sesquiterpene lactones in macrophages correlates with the inhibition of MAP kinases. Hwang D, Fischer NH, Jang BC, Tak H, Kim JK, Lee W Pennington Biomedical Research Center, Louisiana State University, Baton Rouge 70808, USA. PMID: 8831694

Phytochemistry 1995 Jan;38(1):267-70 A biologically active lipophilic flavonol from Tanacetum parthenium. Williams CA, Hoult JR, Harborne JB, Greenham J, Eagles J Department of Botany, School of Plant Sciences, University of Reading, Whiteknights, Berkshire, U.K. PMID: 7766058

Biochem Pharmacol 1992 Jun 9;43(11):2313-20 Inhibition of 5-lipoxygenase and cyclo-oxygenase in leukocytes by feverfew. Involvement of sesquiterpene lactones and other components. Sumner H, Salan U, Knight DW, Hoult JR Pharmacology Group, King's College London, U.K. PMID: 1319159

J Pharm Pharmacol 1990 Aug;42(8):553-7 A comparison of the effects of an extract of feverfew and parthenolide, a component of feverfew, on human platelet activity in-vitro. Groenewegen WA, Heptinstall S Department of Medicine, University Hospital, Nottingham, UK. PMID: 1981582

Ann Rheum Dis 1989 Jul;48(7):547-9 Feverfew in rheumatoid arthritis: a double blind, placebo controlled study. Pattrick M, Heptinstall S, Doherty M Rheumatology Unit, City Hospital, Nottingham. PMID: 2673080

Lancet 1988 Jul 23;2(8604):189-92 Randomised double-blind placebo-controlled trial of feverfew in migraine prevention. Murphy JJ, Heptinstall S, Mitchell JR Department of Medicine, University Hospital, Nottingham. PMID: 2899663

Biomed Biochim Acta 1988;47(10-11):S241-3 Effects of an extract of feverfew (Tanacetum parthenium) on arachidonic acid metabolism in human blood platelets. Loesche W, Groenewegen WA, Krause S, Spangenberg P, Heptinstall S Institute of Pathological Biochemistry, Medical Academy of Erfurt, GDR. PMID: 3248111

Folia Haematol Int Mag Klin Morphol Blutforsch 1988;115(1-2):181-4 Feverfew—an antithrombotic drug? Loesche W, Mazurov AV, Voyno-Yasenetskaya TA, Groenewegen WA, Heptinstall S, Repin VS Institute of Pathological Biochemistry, Medical Academy of Erfurt, GDR. PMID: 2459017

Br Med J (Clin Res Ed) 1985 Aug 31;291(6495):569-73 Efficacy of feverfew as prophylactic treatment of migraine. Johnson ES, Kadam NP, Hylands DM, Hylands PJ PMID: 3929876

Prostaglandins Leukot Med 1982 Jun;8(6):653-60 A platelet phospholipase inhibitor from the medicinal herb feverfew (Tanacetum parthenium). Makheja AN, Bailey JM PMID: 6810384

Chapter Seventeen: Hops

FEBS Lett 2000 Jan 14;465(2-3):103-106 Suppression of cyclooxygenase-2 gene transcription by humulon of beer hop extract studied with reference to glucocorticoid. Yamamoto K, Wang J, Yamamoto S, Tobe H Department of Biochemistry, The University of Tokushima, School of Medicine, Tokushima, Japan [Record supplied by publisher] PMID: 10631313

Food Chem Toxicol 1999 Apr;37(4):271-85 Antiproliferative and cytotoxic effects of prenylated flavonoids from hops (Humulus lupulus) in human cancer cell lines. Miranda CL, Stevens JF, Helmrich A, Henderson MC, Rodriguez RJ, Yang YH, Deinzer ML, Barnes DW, Buhler DR Department of Environmental and Molecular Toxicology, Oregon State University, Corvallis 97331, USA. PMID: 10418944

Leuk Res 1998 Jul;22(7):605-10 Induction of differentiation of myelogenous leukemia cells by humulone, a bitter in the hop. Honma Y, Tobe H, Makishima M, Yokoyama A, Okabe-Kado J Department of Chemotherapy, Saitama Cancer Center Research Institute, Ina, Japan. honma@saitama-cc.go.jp PMID: 9680110

Wien Med Wochenschr 1998;148(13):291-8 [Comparative study for assessing quality of life of patients with exogenous sleep disorders (temporary sleep onset and sleep interruption disorders) treated with a hops-valarian preparation and a benzodiazepine drug]. [Article in German] Schmitz M, Jackel M Institut fur Psychosomatik, Wien. Schmitz@ins.at PMID: 9757514

Biosci Biotechnol Biochem 1997 Jun;61(6):1027-9 Apoptosis to HL-60 by humulone. Tobe H, Kubota M, Yamaguchi M, Kocha T, Aoyagi T Showa College of Pharmaceutical Sciences, Tokyo, Japan. PMID: 9214766

Biosci Biotechnol Biochem 1997 Jan;61(1):158-9 Bone resorption inhibitors from hop extract. Tobe H, Muraki Y, Kitamura K, Komiyama O, Sato Y, Sugioka T, Maruyama HB, Matsuda E, Nagai M Pharma Research and Development Division, Hoechst Japan Limited, Saitama, Japan. PMID: 9028043

Biosci Biotechnol Biochem 1995 Apr;59(4):740-2 Antioxidative activity of hop bitter acids and their analogues. Tagashira M, Watanabe M, Uemitsu N Central Research Laboratories, Asahi Breweries Ltd., Tokyo, Japan. PMID: 7772843

Oncology 1995 Mar-Apr;52(2):156-8 Humulon, a bitter in the hop, inhibits tumor promotion by 12-O-tetradecanoylphorbol-13- acetate in two-stage carcinogenesis in mouse skin. Yasukawa K, Takeuchi M, Takido M College of Pharmacy, Nihon University, Chiba, Japan. PMID: 7854777

J Chromatogr Sci 1992 Oct;30(10):388-91 Fractionation by SFE and microcolumn analysis of the essential oil and the bitter principles of hops. Verschuere M, Sandra P, David F Laboratory of Organic Chemistry, University of Gent, Belgium. PMID: 1430048

Chapter Eighteen: COX-2 Inhibition and Alzheimer's Disease

Phytother Res 1999 Nov;13(7):571-4 Neuroprotective role of curcumin from curcuma longa on ethanol-induced brain damage. Rajakrishnan V, Viswanathan P, Rajasekharan KN, Menon VP Department of Biochemistry, Annamalai University, Annamalai Nagar-608 002, India. PMID 10548748

J Neurosci Res 1999 Aug 1;57(3):295-303 Regional distribution of cyclooxygenase-2 in the hippocampal formation in Alzheimer's disease. Ho L, Pieroni C, Winger D, Purohit DP, Aisen PS, Pasinetti GM Neuroinflammation Research Laboratories of the Department of Psychiatry, The Mount Sinai School of Medicine, New York, New York 10029, USA. gp2@doc.mssm.edu NLM #99341993

J Rheumatol 1999 Apr;26 Suppl 56:25-30 Specific COX-2 inhibitors in arthritis, oncology, and beyond: where is the science headed? Lipsky PE Department of Internal Medicine, The University of Texas Southwestern Medical Center at Dallas, 75235-8884, USA. PMID 10225537

Am J Orthop 1999 Mar;28(3 Suppl):8-12 Role of cyclooxygenase-1 and -2 in health and disease. Lipsky PERheumatic Diseases Division and the Harold C. Simmons Arthritis Research Center, The University of Texas Southwestern Medical Center at Dallas, USA. PMID 10193997

J Photochem Photobiol B 1999 Jan;48(1):63-7 Chemiluminescence determination of the in vivo and in vitro antioxidant activity of RoseOx and carnosic acid. Kuzmenko AI, Morozova RP, Nikolenko IA, Donchenko GV, Richheimer SL, Bailey DT Coenzyme Biochemistry Department, A.V. Palladin Institute of Biochemistry, Ukrainian National Academy of Sciences, Kiev, Ukraine. akuzm@mail.kar.net PMID 10205880

Ukr Biokhim Zh 1999 Jan-Feb;71(1):44-7 Effect of RoseOx on peroxidation of rat mitochondrial lipids. Kuzmenko AI A.V. Palladin Institute of Biochemistry, National Academy of Sciences of Ukraine, Kyiv. [Medline record in process] PMID 10457989

Herbs for Health 1999 Jan/Feb. Dr. James Duke reports at least 6 constitutents can help prevent breakdown of acetylcholine. (Duke- "I'd bet my head of hair that rosemary would have activities parallel to huperzine (FDA approved) and tacrine at retarding the progression of Alzheimers.")

Drugs Exp Clin Res 1999;25(2-3):99-103 Resveratrol, map kinases and neuronal cells: might wine be a neuroprotectant? Tredici G, Miloso M, Nicolini G, Galbiati S, Cavaletti G, Bertelli A Institute of Human Anatomy, Lita Segrate, University of Milan, Italy. gtredici@imiucca.csi.unimi.it PMID 10370870

Crit Rev Neurobiol 1999;13(1):45-82 Cyclooxygenase-2: molecular biology, pharmacology, and neurobiology. O'Banion MK Department of Neurology, University of Rochester School of Medicine and Dentistry, New York 14642, USA. PMID 10223523

J Neurosci Res 1998 Dec 15;54(6):798-804 Beta-amyloid binds to p57NTR and activates NFkappaB in human neuroblastoma cells. Kuner P, Schubenel R, Hertel C F. Hoffmann-LaRoche AG, Pharma Division Preclinical Research, Basel, Switzerland. PMID 9856863

J Nat Prod 1998 Sep;61(9):1090-5 Anti-AIDS agents. 30. Anti-HIV activity of oleanolic acid, pomolic acid, and structurally related triterpenoids. Kashiwada Y, Wang HK, Nagao T, Kitanaka S, Yasuda I, Fujioka T, Yamagishi T, Cosentino LM, Kozuka M, Okabe H, Ikeshiro Y, Hu CQ, Yeh E, Lee KH Natural Products Laboratory, Division of Medicinal Chemistry and Natural Products, School of Pharmacy, University of North Carolina, Chapel Hill, North Carolina 27599, USA. PMID 9748372

Proc Natl Acad Sci U S A 1998 Sep 1;95(18):10954-9 Cyclooxygenase-2 inhibition prevents delayed death of CA1 hippocampal neurons following global ischemia. Nakayama M, Uchimura K, Zhu RL, Nagayama T, Rose ME, Stetler RA, Isakson PC, Chen J, Graham SH Department of Neurology, University of Pittsburgh, Pittsburgh, PA 15213, USA. NLM #98393752

Cancer Res 1998 Jun 1;58(11):2323-7 Antioxidants reduce cyclooxygenase-2 expression, prostaglandin production, and proliferation in colorectal cancer cells. Chinery R, Beauchamp RD, Shyr Y, Kirkland SC, Coffey RJ, Morrow JD Department of Medicine, The Vanderbilt Cancer Center, Vanderbilt University Medical Center, Nashville, Tennessee 37232, USA.

Neurology 1998 Apr;50(4):986-90 Nonsteroidal anti-inflammatory drug use and Alzheimer-type pathology in aging. Mackenzie IR, Munoz DG Department of Pathology and Laboratory Medicine, Vancouver General Hospital, British Columbia, Canada. NLM #98226034

Cancer Res 1998 Feb 15;58(4):717-23 Novel triterpenoids suppress inducible nitric oxide synthase (iNOS) and inducible cyclooxygenase (COX-2) in mouse macrophages. Suh N, Honda T, Finlay HJ, Barchowsky A, Williams C, Benoit NE, Xie QW, Nathan C, Gribble GW, Sporn MB Department of Pharmacology and Norris Cotton Cancer Center, Dartmouth Medical School, Hanover, New Hampshire 03755, USA. PMID 9485026

Mol Chem Neuropathol 1998 Feb;33(2):139-48 Oxidized lipoproteins may play a role in neuronal cell death in Alzheimer disease. Draczynska-Lusiak B, Doung A, Sun AY Department of Pharmacology, University of Missouri, Columbia 65212, USA. PMID 9565971

Arch Toxicol Suppl 1998;20:227-36 Development of in vitro models for cellular and molecular studies in toxicology and chemoprevention. Mace K, Offord EA, Harris CC, Pfeifer AM Nestle Research Center, Lausanne, Switzerland. PMID 9442296

Annu Rev Pharmacol Toxicol 1998;38:97-120 Cyclooxygenases 1 and 2. Vane JR, Bakhle YS, Botting RM William Harvey Research Institute, St Bartholomew's, London, United Kingdom. PMID 9597150

Int J Tissue React 1998;20(1):3-15 Mechanism of action of antiinflammatory drugs. Vane JR, Botting RM William Harvey Research Institute, St Bartholomew's, UK. PMID 9561441

J Neurosci Res 1997 Dec 15;50(6):937-45 Cyclooxygenase 2 RNA message abundance, stability, and hypervariability in sporadic Alzheimer neocortex. Lukiw WJ, Bazan NG Neuroscience Center of Excellence, Louisiana State University School of Medicine, LSU Medical Center, New Orleans 70112-2272, USA. wluki@lsumc.edu PMID 98112387

Prostaglandins 1997 Sep; 54(3):601-24 Cyclooxygenases and the central nervous system. Kaufmann WE, Andreasson KI, Isakson PC,Worley PF, Department of Pathology, Johns Hopkins University of Medicine, Baltimore, MD, USA. PMID 9373877

Eur J Pharmacol 1997 Sep 3;334(1):103-5 Effect of selected triterpenoids on chronic dermal inflammation. Manez S, Recio MC, Giner RM, Rios JL Departament de Farmacologia, Universitat de Valencia, Spain. PMID 9346335 Exp Gerontol 1997 Jul-Oct;32(4-5):431-40 The nitric oxide hypothesis of brain aging. McCann SM Pennington Biomedical Research Center, Louisiana State University, Baton Rouge 70808-4124, USA. PMID 9315447

Cancer Lett 1997 Jan 1;111(1-2):7-13 Effects of oleanolic acid and ursolic acid on inhibiting tumor growth and enhancing the recovery of hematopoietic system postirradiation in mice. Hsu HY, Yang JJ, Lin CC Department of Radiotherapy, Kaohsiung Medical College, Taiwan, ROC. PMID 9022122

Cancer Lett 1996 Jun 24;104(1):43-8 Inhibition by rosemary and carnosol of 7,12-dimethylbenz[a]anthracene (DMBA)-induced rat mammary tumorigenesis and in vivo DMBA-DNA adduct formation. Singletary K, MacDonald C, Wallig M Department of Food Science and Human Nutrition, University of Illinois, Urbana 61801, USA. PMID 8640744

Cancer Res 1996 May 15;56(10):2281-4 Anti-invasive activity of ursolic acid correlates with the reduced expression of matrix metalloproteinase-9 (MMP-9) in HT1080 human fibrosarcoma cells. Cha HJ, Bae SK, Lee HY, Lee OH, Sato H, Seiki M, Park BC, Kim KW Department of Molecular Biology, Pusan National University, Korea. PMID 8625299

Food Chem Toxicol 1996 May;34(5):449-56 An evaluation of the antioxidant and antiviral action of extracts of rosemary and Provencal herbs. Aruoma OI, Spencer JP, Rossi R, Aeschbach R, Khan A, Mahmood N, Munoz A, Murcia A, Butler J, Halliwell B Pharmacology Group, University of London King's College, UK. PMID 8655093

Neurology 1996 Mar;46(3):707-19 Cerebral amyloid deposition and diffuse plaques in «normal» aging: Evidence for presymptomatic and very mild Alzheimer's disease. Morris JC, Storandt M, McKeel DW Jr, Rubin EH, Price JL, Grant EA, Berg L Alzheimer's Disease Research Center, Department of Neurology, Washington University School of Medicine, St. Louis, M0 63110, USA PMID 96173680

Anticancer Res 1996 Jan-Feb;16(1):481-6 MCF-7 cell cycle arrested at G1 through ursolic acid, and increased reduction of tetrazolium salts. Es-Saady D, Simon A, Jayat-Vignoles C, Chulia AJ, Delage C Faculte de Pharmacie, Limoges, France. PMID 8615658

J Ethnopharmacol 1995 Dec 1;49(2):57-68 Pharmacology of oleanolic acid and ursolic acid. Liu J Department of Pharmacology, Toxicology and Therapeutics, University of Kansas Medical Center, Kansas City 66160-7417, USA. PMID 8847885

Cancer Lett 1995 Sep 4;96(1):23-9 Effects of three dietary phytochemicals from tea, rosemary and turmeric on inflammation-induced nitrite production. Chan MM, Ho CT, Huang HI Department of Biological Sciences, Rutgers, State University of New Jersey, Piscataway 08855-1059, USA. PMID 7553604

Carcinogenesis 1995 Sep;16(9):2057-62 Rosemary components inhibit benzo[a]pyrene-induced genotoxicity in human bronchial cells. Offord EA, Mace K, Ruffieux C, Malnoe A, Pfeifer AM Nestle Research Centre, Lausanne, Switzerland. PMID 7554054

Cancer Lett 1995 Aug 1;94(2):213-8 Anti-angiogenic activity of triterpene acids. Sohn KH, Lee HY, Chung HY, Young HS, Yi SY, Kim KW Department of Molecular Biology, Pusan National University, Korea. PMID 7543366

Planta Med 1995 Aug;61(4):333-6 Inhibition of lipid peroxidation and superoxide generation by diterpenoids from Rosmarinus officinalis. Haraguchi H, Saito T, Okamura N, Yagi A Faculty of Engineering, Fukuyama University, Japan. PMID 7480180

Chung Kuo Yao Li Hsueh Pao 1995 Mar;16(2):97-102 Protective effect of oleanolic acid against chemical-induced acute necrotic liver injury in mice. Liu J, Liu Y, Klaassen CD Department of Pharmacology, Toxicology and Therapeutics, University of Kansas Medical Center, Kansas City 66160-7417, USA. PMID 7597924

Yao Hsueh Hsueh Pao 1995;30(2):98-102 [Effects of berberine on platelet aggregation and plasma levels of TXB2 and 6-keto-PGF1 alpha in rats with reversible middle cerebral artery occlusion].[Article in Chinese] Wu JF, Liu TP Department of Pharmacology, Nanjing Medical University. PMID 7785438

Cancer Res 1994 Feb 1;54(3):701-8 Inhibition of skin tumorigenesis by rosemary and its constituents carnosol and ursolic acid. Huang MT, Ho CT, Wang ZY, Ferraro T, Lou YR, Stauber K, Ma W, Georgiadis C, Laskin JD, Conney AH Department of Chemical Biology and Pharmacognosy, College of Pharmacy, Rutgers, State University of New Jersey, Piscataway 08855-0789. PMID 8306331

J Pharmacol Exp Ther 1993 Sep;266(3):1607-13 Protective effects of oleanolic acid on acetaminophen-induced hepatotoxicity in mice. Liu J, Liu Y, Madhu C, Klaassen CD Department of Pharmacology, Toxicology and Therapeutics, University of Kansas Medical Center, Kansas City. PMID 8371159

J Nat Prod 1993 Aug;56(8):1426-30 Corrected] [published erratum appears in J Nat Prod 1994 Apr;57(4):552 Inhibitory effect of carnosic acid on HIV-1 protease in cell-free assays. Paris A, Strukelj B, Renko M, Turk V, Pukl M, Umek A, Korant BD Department of Biochemistry, Jozef Stefan Institute, Ljubljana, Slovenia. PMID 8229021

Mutat Res 1992 Oct;269(2):193-200 Natural antioxidants as inhibitors of oxygen species induced mutagenicity. Minnunni M, Wolleb U, Mueller O, Pfeifer A, Aeschbacher HU Nestec Ltd, Nestle Research Centre, Vers-chez-les-Blanc, Lausanne, Switzerland. PMID 1383702

J Pharm Pharmacol 1992 May;44(5):456-8 Anti-inflammatory activity of oleanolic acid in rats and mice. Singh GB, Singh S, Bani S, Gupta BD, Banerjee SK Pharmacology Department, Regional Research Laboratory, Jammu-Tawi, India. PMID 1359067

FEBS Lett 1992 Mar 16;299(3):213-7 Characterization of ursolic acid as a lipoxygenase and cyclooxygenase inhibitor using macrophages, platelets and differentiated HL60 leukemic cells. Najid A, Simon A, Cook J, Chable-Rabinovitch H, Delage C, Chulia AJ, Rigaud M CJF INSERM 88-03, Faculte de Medecine, Universite de Limoges, France. PMID 1544497

Biochem Pharmacol 1991 Oct 9;42(9):1673-81 Inhibition of mammalian 5-lipoxygenase and cyclo-oxygenase by flavonoids and phenolic dietary additives. Relationship to antioxidant activity and to iron ion-reducing ability. Laughton MJ, Evans PJ, Moroney MA, Hoult JR, Halliwell B Department of Biochemistry, King's College London, U.K. 1656994

Biochem Int 1991 Jul;24(5):981-90 Protective effect of oleanolic acid and ursolic acid against lipid peroxidation. Balanehru S, Nagarajan B Department of Microbiology & Tumor Biochemistry, Cancer Institute, Madras, India. PMID 1776961

Cancer Lett 1986 Dec;33(3):279-85 Inhibitory effects of ursolic and oleanolic acid on skin tumor promotion by 12-O-tetradecanoylphorbol-13-acetate. Tokuda H, Ohigashi H, Koshimizu K, Ito Y PMID 3802058

Chapter Nineteen: Free-Radical Damage and Alzheimer's Disease

J Neuropathol Exp Neurol 1999 Aug;58(8):803-14 Alzheimer disease: curly fibers and tangles in organs other than brain. Miklossy J, Taddei K, Martins R, Escher G, Kraftsik R, Pillevuit O, Lepori D, Campiche M PMID: 10446805, UI: 99374471

Neuroreport 1999 Jun 23;10(9):1889-91 Long-term intracerebral inflammatory response after experimental focal brain injury in rat. Holmin S, Mathiesen T PMID: 10501527, UI: 99429635

Exp Gerontol 1999 Jun;34(3):453-61 The importance of inflammatory mechanisms for the development of Alzheimer's disease. Eikelenboom P, Veerhuis R PMID: 10433400, UI: 99360782

Ann Pharmacother 1999 Apr;33(4):441-50 Cholinesterase inhibitors: a therapeutic strategy for Alzheimer disease. Krall WJ, Sramek JJ, Cutler NR PMID: 10332536, UI: 99264940

J Leukoc Biol 1999 Apr;65(4):409-15 Inflammation of the brain in Alzheimer's disease: implications for therapy. McGeer PL, McGeer EG PMID: 10204568, UI: 99219262

Am J Orthop 1999 Mar;28(3 Suppl):8-12 Role of cyclooxygenase-1 and -2 in health and disease. Lipsky PE PMID: 10193997, UI: 99208340

Brain Res 1998 Oct 5;807(1-2):110-7 Alzheimer's beta-amyloid peptides induce inflammatory cascade in human vascular cells: the roles of cytokines and CD40. Suo Z, Tan J, Placzek A, Crawford F, Fang C, Mullan M PMID: 9757011, UI: 98432082

Curr Pharm Des 1998 Aug;4(4):335-48 Therapeutic approaches to the treatment of neuroinflammatory diseases. Hays SJ PMID: 10197047, UI: 99212796

J Neurochem 1998 Feb;70(2):699-707 Inflammatory signals induce neurotrophin expression in human microglial cells. Heese K, Hock C, Otten U PMID: 9453564, UI: 98114309

Brain Pathol 1998 Jan;8(1):65-72 Glial-neuronal interactions in Alzheimer's disease: the potential role of a 'cytokine cycle' in disease progression. Griffin WS, Sheng JG, Royston MC, Gentleman SM, McKenzie JE, Graham DI, Roberts GW, Mrak RE PMID: 9458167, UI: 98117371

J Geriatr Psychiatry Neurol 1998 Winter;11(4):163-73 Complementary and alternative medicines for Alzheimer's disease. Ott BR, Owens NJ PMID: 10230994, UI: 99246025

Acta Medica (Hradec Kralove) 1998;41(4):155-7 Huperzine A—an interesting anticholinesterase compound from the Chinese herbal medicine. Patocka J PMID: 9951045, UI: 99136196

Tijdschr Gerontol Geriatr 1997 Oct;28(5):213-8 [Inflammatory mechanisms in the pathogenesis of Alzheimer's disease]. [Article in Dutch] Verbeek MM, Otte-Holler I, Ruiter DJ, de Waal RM PMID: 9526791, UI: 98187539

Crit Rev Biochem Mol Biol 1997;32(5):361-404 A beta amyloidogenesis: unique, or variation on a systemic theme? Kisilevsky R, Fraser PE PMID: 9383610, UI: 98044867

Brain Res Brain Res Rev 1995 Sep;21(2):195-218 The inflammatory response system of brain: implications for therapy of Alzheimer and other neurodegenerative diseases. McGeer PL, McGeer EG PMID: 8866675, UI: 97020290

Chapter Twenty: Other Phytochemical Strategies for Dealing with Brain Plaque and Related COX-2 Inflammation

J Neurochem 1999 Jun;72(6):2601-9 Oxidized low-density lipoprotein induces neuronal death: implications for calcium, reactive oxygen species, and caspases. Keller JN, Hanni KB, Markesbery WR PMID: 10349872

J Pharm Pharmacol 1999 May;51(5):527-34 Medicinal plants and Alzheimer's disease: from ethnobotany to phytotherapy. Perry EK, Pickering AT, Wang WW, Houghton PJ, Perry NS PMID: 10411211

Free Radic Biol Med 1999 May;26(9-10):1346-55 Neuroinflammatory processes are important in neurodegenerative diseases: an hypothesis to explain the increased formation of reactive oxygen and nitrogen species as major factors involved in neurodegenerative disease development. Floyd RA PMID: 10381209

Phytother Res 1999 Feb;13(1):50-4 Asiaticoside-induced elevation of antioxidant levels in healing wounds. Shukla A, Rasik AM, Dhawan BN Pharmacology Department, Central Drug Research Institute, Lucknow, India. gshukla@zoo.uvm.edu PMID 10189951

Brain Pathol 1999 Jan;9(1):133-46 Oxidative alterations in Alzheimer's disease. Markesbery WR, Carney JM PMID: 9989456

J Clin Endocrinol Metab 1999 Jan;84(1):323-7 Decreased melatonin levels in postmortem cerebrospinal fluid in relation to aging, Alzheimer's disease, and apolipoprotein E-epsilon4/4 genotype. Liu RY, Zhou JN, van Heerikhuize J, Hofman MA, Swaab DF Netherlands Institute for Brain Research, Amsterdam. PMID: 9920102, UI: 99116830

Proceedings of the National Academy of Sciences 1999;96 Brahmi

Exp Neurol 1998 Nov;154(1):89-98 Inflammation and Alzheimer's disease: relationships between pathogenic mechanisms and clinical expression. Eikelenboom P, Rozemuller JM, van Muiswinkel FL PMID: 9875271

Front Biosci 1998 Apr 16;3:d436-46 The essential role of inflammation and induced gene expression in the pathogenic pathway of Alzheimer's disease. Nilsson L, Rogers J, Potter H PMID: 9545438

Neurology 1998 Apr;50(4):986-90 Nonsteroidal anti-inflammatory drug use and Alzheimer-type pathology in aging. Mackenzie IR, Munoz DG PMID: 9566383

J Neural Transm Suppl 1998;54:159-66 Mechanisms of cell death in Alzheimer disease—immunopathology. McGeer PL, McGeer EG PMID: 9850924

CMAJ 1997 Apr 1;156(7):1040-2 Amyloid beta protein and Alzheimer disease. Square D PMID: 9099177

J Am Geriatr Soc 1996 Jul;44(7):865-70 Is there a role for estrogen replacement therapy in the prevention and treatment of dementia? Birge SJ PMID: 8675940

Neurology 1996 Feb;46(2):425-9 Prospective neuropsychological assessment of nondemented patients with biopsy proven senile plaques. Mackenzie IR, McLachlan RS, Kubu CS, Miller LA Department of Pathology, University Hospital, London, Ontario, Canada. PMID: 8614506

Chapter Twenty-One: Omega-3—A Complement to Herbal Inhibition of Inflammatory COX-2

Int J Oncol 1999 Nov;15(5):1011-1015 Antiangiogenicity of docosahexaenoic acid and its role in the suppression of breast cancer cell growth in nude mice. Rose DP, Connolly JM Division of Nutrition and Endocrinology, American Health Foundation, Valhalla, NY 10595, USA. PMID: 10536186

Pharmacol Res 1999 Sep;40(3):211-25 Health benefits of docosahexaenoic acid. Horrocks LA, Yeo YK Docosa Foods Ltd, 1275 Kinnear Road, Columbus, OH, 43212-1155, USA, [Medline record in process] PMID: 10479465

Med Hypotheses 1999 Aug;53(2):172-4 Weight loss in cancer and Alzheimer's disease is mediated by a similar pathway. Knittweis J Research Solutions, Philadelphia, PA, USA. PMID: 10532714

Ann Med 1999 Aug;31(4):282-7 Dietary fatty acids and allergy. Kankaanpaa P, Sutas Y, Salminen S, Lichtenstein A, Isolauri E Department of Biochemistry and Food Chemistry, University of Turku, Finland. si.kankaanpaa@utu.fi PMID: 10480759

Eur J Cancer Prev 1999 Jul;8(3):213-21 Possible beneficial effect of fish and fish n-3 polyunsaturated fatty acids in breast and colorectal cancer. de Deckere EA Unilever Nutrition Centre, Unilever Research Vlaardingen, The Netherlands. PMID: 10443950

Carcinogenesis 1999 Feb;20(2):249-54 Fish oil constituent docosahexa-enoic acid selectively inhibits growth of human papillomavirus immortalized keratinocytes. Chen D, Auborn K Long Island Jewish Medical Center, The Long Island Campus for Albert Einstein College of Medicine, Department of Otolaryngology, New Hyde Park, NY 11040, USA. PMID: 10069461

Drugs 1998 Apr;55(4):487-96 Lipid mediators in inflammatory disorders. Heller A, Koch T, Schmeck J, van Ackern K Department of Anaesthesiology and Intensive Care Medicine, University of Dresden, Germany. heller@rumms.uni-mannheim.de PMID: 9561339

Fats that Heal, Fats that Kill Erasmus, U.; Alive Books 1999

Am J Epidemiol 1998 Feb 15;147(4):342-52 Adipose tissue omega-3 and omega-6 fatty acid content and breast cancer in the EURAMIC study. European Community Multicenter Study on Antioxidants, Myocardial Infarction, and Breast Cancer. Simonsen N, van't Veer P, Strain JJ, Martin-Moreno JM, Huttunen JK, Navajas JF, Martin BC, Thamm M, Kardinaal AF, Kok FJ, Kohlmeier L University of North Carolina, Chapel Hill 27599, USA.

Cancer Lett 1998 Feb 13;124(1):1-7 Alteration of murine mammary tumorigenesis by dietary enrichment with n-3 fatty acids in fish oil. Hubbard NE, Lim D, Erickson KL Department of Cell Biology and Human Anatomy, University of California, School of Medicine, Davis 95616-8643, USA. nehubbard@ucdavis.edu PMID: 9500184

Cancer 1998 Jan 15;82(2):395-402 Dietary omega-3 polyunsaturated fatty acids plus vitamin E restore immunodeficiency and prolong survival for severely ill patients with generalized malignancy: a randomized control trial. Gogos CA, Ginopoulos P, Salsa B, Apostolidou E, Zoumbos NC, Kalfarentzos F Department of Medicine, Patras University Medical School, Rion-Patras, Greece. PMID: 9445198

Eur J Cancer Prev 1997 Dec;6(6):540-9 Dietary fat intake and risk of lung cancer: a prospective study of 51,452 Norwegian men and women. Veierod MB, Laake P, Thelle DS Section for Medical Statistics, University of Oslo, Blindern, Norway.

Free Radic Res 1997 Dec;27(6):591-7 Fish oil and oxidative stress by inflammatory leukocytes. Carbonell T, Rodenas J, Miret S, Mitjavila MT Department of Physiology, Faculty of Biology, University of Barcelona, Spain. PMID 9455694

Cancer Res 1997 Aug 15;57(16):3465-70 Dietary fat and colon cancer: modulation of cyclooxygenase-2 by types and amount of dietary fat during the postinitiation stage of colon carcinogenesis. Singh J, Hamid R, Reddy BS Division of Nutritional Carcinogenesis, American Health Foundation, Valhalla, New York 10595, USA. PMID: 9270014

Lipids 1997 Mar;32(3):293-302 Incorporation of long-chain n-3 fatty acids in tissues and enhanced bone marrow cellularity with docosahexaenoic acid feeding in post-weanling Fischer 344 rats. Atkinson TG, Barker HJ, Meckling-Gill KA Department of Human Biology and Nutritional Sciences, University of Guelph, Ontario, Canada. PMID: 9076666

Am J Epidemiol 1997 Jan 1;145(1):33-41 Polyunsaturated fatty acids, antioxidants, and cognitive function in very old men. Kalmijn S, Feskens EJ, Launer LJ, Kromhout D Department of Chronic Diseases and Environmental Epidemiology, National Institute of Public Health and the Environment, Bilthoven, The Netherlands. PMID: 8982020

J Nutr 1996 Jun;126(6):1515-33 Modulation of inflammation and cytokine production by dietary (n-3) fatty acids. Blok WL, Katan MB, van der Meer JW Department of General Internal Medicine, University Hospital Nijmegen, Nijmegen, The Netherlands. PMID: 8648424

Lipids 1996 Mar;31 Suppl:S243-7 Effects of modulation of inflammatory and immune parameters in patients with rheumatic and inflammatory disease receiving dietary supplementation of n-3 and n-6 fatty acids. Kremer JM Division of Rheumatology, Albany Medical College, New York 12208, USA. PMID: 8729127

Cancer Epidemiol Biomarkers Prev 1996 Feb;5(2):115-9 Correlation between biomarkers of omega-3 fatty acid consumption and questionnaire data in African American and Caucasian United States males with and without prostatic carcinoma. Godley PA, Campbell MK, Miller C, Gallagher P, Martinson FE, Mohler JL, Sandler RS Division of Hematology/Oncology, University of North Carolina at Chapel Hill 27599-7305, USA. PMID: 8850272

Med Hypotheses 1996 Feb;46(2):107-15 Fish oil may impede tumour angiogenesis and invasiveness by down-regulating protein kinase C and modulating eicosanoid production. McCarty MF Nutrition 21, San Diego, CA 92109, USA. PMID: 8692033

Nutrition 1996 Jan;12(1 Suppl):S39-42 Dietary omega-3 polyunsaturated fats and breast cancer. Cave WT Jr Endocrine Unit, University of Rochester School of Medicine, New York, USA. PMID: 8850219

Br J Cancer 1996 Jan;73(1):36-43 Dietary fish oil (MaxEPA) enhances pancreatic carcinogenesis in azaserine-treated rats. Appel MJ, Woutersen RA TNO Nutrition and Food Research Institute, Department of Pathology, Zeist, The Netherlands. PMID: 8554980

Nutrition 1996 Jan;12(1 Suppl):S2-4 Historical perspective and potential use of n-3 fatty acids in therapy of cancer cachexia. Karmali RA Bryan Cave, New York, New York, USA. PMID: 8850210

Adv Exp Med Biol 1996;399:87-94 Metabolism of exogenous and endogenous arachidonic acid in cancer. Phinney SD Department of Internal Medicine, University of California at Davis 95616, USA. PMID: 8937550

Eur J Clin Invest 1995 Dec;25(12):915-9 Omega-3 fatty acids suppress the enhanced production of 5-lipoxygenase products from polymorph neutrophil granulocytes in cystic fibrosis. Keicher U, Koletzko B, Reinhardt D Kinderpoliklinik, Ludwig-Maximilians-Universitat, Munich, Germany. PMID: 8719931

Proc Soc Exp Biol Med 1995 Dec;210(3):227-33 Omega-3 fatty acid-containing liposomes in cancer therapy. Jenski LJ, Zerouga M, Stillwell W Department of Biology, Indiana University-Purdue University at Indianapolis 46303-5132, USA. PMID: 8539260

302

Infusionsther Transfusionsmed 1995 Oct;22(5):280-4 Benefits of early postoperative enteral feeding in cancer patients. Braga M, Vignali A, Gianotti L, Cestari A, Profili M, Di Carlo V Department of Surgery, Scientific Institute San Raffaele, University of Milan, Italy. PMID: 8924741

Eur J Cancer Prev 1995 Aug;4(4):329-32 Fish, n-3 fatty acids and human colorectal and breast cancer mortality. Caygill CP, Hill MJ Public Health Laboratory Service, Communicable Disease Surveillance Centre, Colindale, London, UK. PMID: 7549825

Cancer Pract 1995 Jul-Aug;3(4):239-46 Effect of major dietary modifications on immune system in patients with breast cancer: a pilot study. Garritson BK, Nikaein A, Peters GN, Gorman MA, King CC, Liepa GU PMID: 7620489

Oncology 1995 Jul-Aug;52(4):265-71 The role of fatty acids and eicosanoid synthesis inhibitors in breast carcinoma. Noguchi M, Rose DP, Earashi M, Miyazaki I Department of Surgery (II), Kanazawa University Hospital, School of Medicine, Japan. PMID: 7777237

Oncology 1995 Jul-Aug;52(4):265-71 The role of fatty acids and eicosanoid synthesis inhibitors in breast carcinoma. Noguchi M, Rose DP, Earashi M, Miyazaki I Department of Surgery (II), Kanazawa University Hospital, School of Medicine, Japan. PMID: 7777237

J Natl Cancer Inst 1995 Apr 19;87(8):587-92 Influence of diets containing eicosapentaenoic or docosahexaenoic acid on growth and metastasis of breast cancer cells in nude mice. Rose DP, Connolly JM, Rayburn J, Coleman M Division of Nutrition and Endocrinology, American Health Foundation, Vallhalla, N.Y. 10595, USA. PMID: 7752256

Cancer Detect Prev 1995;19(5):415-7 The effect of dietary omega-3 polyunsaturated fatty acids on T-lymphocyte subsets of patients with solid tumors. Gogos CA, Ginopoulos P, Zoumbos NC, Apostolidou E, Kalfarentzos F Department of Medicine, Patras University, Medical School, Greece. PMID: 7585727

Arterioscler Thromb 1994 Nov;14(11):1829-36 The omega-3 fatty acid docosahexaenoate reduces cytokine-induced expression of proatherogenic and proinflammatory proteins in human endothelial cells. De Caterina R, Cybulsky MI, Clinton SK, Gimbrone MA Jr, Libby P Department of Medicine, Brigham and Women's Hospital, Harvard Medical School, Boston, Mass 02115. PMID: 7524649

Biochim Biophys Acta 1994 Nov 10;1224(2):255-63 Role of capsaicin, curcumin and dietary n-3 fatty acids in lowering the generation of reactive oxygen species in rat peritoneal macrophages. Joe B, Lokesh BR Department of Biochemistry and Nutrition, Central Food Technological Research Institute, Mysore, India. PMID: 7981240

Anticancer Res 1994 May-Jun;14(3A):1145-54 Omega-3 fatty acids can improve radioresponse modifying tumor interstitial pressure, blood rheology and membrane peroxidability. Baronzio G, Freitas I, Griffini P, Bertone V, Pacini F, Mascaro G, Razzini E, Gramaglia A Surgery Unit, USL 71, Cuggiono, Italy. PMID: 8074465

Ann Nutr Metab 1994;38(6):349-58 Studies on anti-inflammatory activity of spice principles and dietary n-3 polyunsaturated fatty acids on carrageenan-induced inflammation in rats. Reddy AC, Lokesh BR Department of Biochemistry and Nutrition, Central Food Technological Research Institute, Mysore, India. PMID: 7702364

Gastroenterology 1993 Nov;105(5):1317-22 Effects of fish oil on rectal cell proliferation, mucosal fatty acids, and prostaglandin E2 release in healthy subjects. Bartram HP, Gostner A, Scheppach W, Reddy BS, Rao CV, Dusel G, Richter F, Richter A, Kasper H Department of Medicine, University of Wurzburg, Germany. PMID: 8224635

Lipids 1993 Feb;28(2):103-8 Docosahexaenoic acid increases permeability of lipid vesicles and tumor cells. Stillwell W, Ehringer W, Jenski LJ Department of Biology, Indiana University-Purdue University, Indianapolis 46202-5132. PMID: 8441334

Immunol Lett 1992 Sep;34(1):13-7 Dietary supplementation with fish oil enhances in vivo synthesis of tumor necrosis factor. Chang HR, Arsenijevic D, Pechere JC, Piguet PF, Mensi N, Girardier L, Dulloo AG Department of Genetics and Microbiology, University of Geneva Medical School, Switzerland. PMID: 1478702

Gastroenterology 1992 Sep;103(3):883-91 Effect of omega-3 fatty acids on rectal mucosal cell proliferation in subjects at risk for colon cancer. Anti M, Marra G, Armelao F, Bartoli GM, Ficarelli R, Percesepe A, De Vitis I, Maria G, Sofo L, Rapaccini GL, et al Department of Internal Medicine, Catholic University of Rome, Italy. PMID: 1386825

Ann Intern Med 1992 Apr 15;116(8):609-14 Dietary supplementation with fish oil in ulcerative colitis. Stenson WF, Cort D, Rodgers J, Burakoff R, DeSchryver-Kecskemeti K, Gramlich TL, Beeken W Jewish Hospital of St. Louis, Missouri 63110. PMID: 1312317

Am J Gastroenterol 1992 Apr;87(4):432-7 Fish oil fatty acid supplementation in active ulcerative colitis: a double-blind, placebo-controlled, crossover study. Aslan A, Triadafilopoulos G Gastroenterology Section, Veterans Affairs Medical Center, Martinez, California. PMID: 1553930

J Nutr Sci Vitaminol (Tokyo) 1992;Spec No:148-52 n-3 fatty acids: biochemical actions in cancer. Karmali R Memorial Sloan-Kettering Cancer Center, New York, New York. PMID: 1297728

Br J Cancer 1991 Dec;64(6):1157-60 Essential fatty acid distribution in the plasma and tissue phospholipids of patients with benign and malignant prostatic disease. Chaudry A, McClinton S, Moffat LE, Wahle KW Department of Urology, Aberdeen Royal Infirmary, UK. PMID: 1764380

Rheum Dis Clin North Am 1991 May;17(2):373-89 Dietary omega-3 fatty acids: effects on lipid mediators of inflammation and rheumatoid arthritis. Sperling RI Department of Medicine, Harvard Medical School, Boston, Massachusetts. PMID: 1862246

Nutr Cancer 1989;12(1):61-8 Fish consumption and breast cancer risk: an ecological study. Kaizer L, Boyd NF, Kriukov V, Tritchler D Ludwig Institute for Cancer Research (Toronto Branch), Ontario, Canada. PMID: 2710648

J Nutr 1989 Apr;119(4):521-8 Summary of the NATO advanced research workshop on dietary omega 3 and omega 6 fatty acids: biological effects and nutritional essentiality. Simopoulos AP Division of Nutritional Sciences, International Life Sciences Institute Research Foundation. PMID: 2564887

Chapter Twenty-Two: Alternative Delivery Systems of Herbal COX-2 Inhibitors: Transdermal Herbalism and Aromatherapy

J Essent Oil Res. 1997 9: 53-56 Effect of essential oils on the retina in the aging rat: a possibletherapeutic effect. Recsan Z, Pagliuca G, Piretti M V et al.

PhytotherRes. 1996 10: 551-554 Antifungal activity of lemongrass oil and lemongrass oil cream. Wannisorn B, Jarikasem S, Soontorntanasart T..

Acta Manilana 1995. 43. 19-23. Screening for the antibacterial activity of essential oils from the Philippine plants. Ontengco D, Dayap LA, Capal T V.

Indian J Malariol. 1995 32: 104-111 Relative efficacy ofvarious oils in repelling mosquitoes. Ansari M A, Razdan R K.

The Aromatherapy Practitioner Reference Manual 1995 Vol 2. p516 Sheppard-Hangar S., Atlantic Institute of Aromatherapy.

Aromatherapy for Health Professionals Price S., Churchill Livingstone, 1995

Essential Oil Safety Tisserand R & Balacs T., Churchill Livingstone, 1995

Indian J Pharmaceut Sci. 1994 56 (6)227-231 Screening of some Essential Oils against Ringworm fungi. Yadav P, Dubey N K.

Plant Aromatics Watts M., The Atlantic Institute of Aromatherapy, Tampa, Florida 1994

Potters New Cyclopedia of Botanical Drugs &Preparations Wren RC, Saffron Walden 1994

Journal of Agriculture & Food Chemistry. 1993 Feb, Vol 41, No 2. Potential anticarcinogenic natural products isolated from Lemongrass Oil. Zheng G, Kenney P M, Lamm K T.

Critical Reviews in Food Science and Nutrition. 33 (1) 57-62. 1993. Psychophysiological Effect of Odor. Manley C.

Journal of Canadian Pharmacology 1993;126 10: 503-504. R Locok Phytother Res. 1992 5 (5) 279-281 An Evaluation of the toxicity of the oils of Cymbopogon citratus and Citrusmedica in Rats. Mishra A K, Kishore N, Dubey N K.

Ethonopharmacology. 1991 Aug 34(1) 43-8. Myrcene mimics the peripheral analgesic activity of lemongrass tea. Lorenzetti B, Souza G, Sarti S, Santon FD, Ferreira S.

American Journal of Psychiatry 1991 Mar;148(3):374-5 Transdermal nicotine and smoking behavior in psychiatric patients. Hartman N, Leong GB, Glynn SM, Wilkins JN, Jarvik ME.

Chem Senses. 16: 183 1991 Effect of odors on cardiac response patterns in a reaction time task. Kikuchi A, Tanida M, Uemoyama S, Abe T, Yamaguchi H.

Chem Senses. 1991 16: 198 Effects of odors on humans (11) Reducing effects of mental stress and fatigue. Nagai H, Nakagawa M, Nakamura M, Fujii W, Inui T, Asakura Y.

Out of the Earth Mills S., London: Viking, 1991

Lancet 1990 Aug 4;336(8710):265-9 Effects of transdermal versus oral hormone replacement therapy on bone density in spine and proximal femur in postmenopausal women. Stevenson JC, Cust MP, Gangar KF, Hillard TC, Lees B, Whitehead MI.

Dermatologica 1990;180(1):36-9 Percutaneous absorption of zinc from zinc oxide applied topically to intact skin in man. Agren MS.

J Toxicol Clin Exp. 1990 10. (6) 361-373 Amoebicidal effect of essential oils in vitro. de Blasi V, Debrot S, Menoud P A, Gendre L, Schowing J.

Chemical Abstracts. 1990 Vol 114. Anti viral compositions containing proanthocyanidols. Application for patent. Cariel L & Jean D.

Pharmazie in Unsererzeit 1989 May;18(3):82-6 [Skin absorption of volatile oils. Pharmacokinetics] Hautdurchdringung atherischer Ole. Weyers W, Brodbeck R. Pharmakokinetische Untersuchungen.

International Journal for Vitamin and Nutrition Research 1989;59(4):333-7 Dermal penetration and systemic distribution of 14C-labeled vitamin E in human skin grafted athymic nude mice. Klain GJ.

LIPIDS vol 24, No 8(1989). Impact of Lemongrass on serum cholesterol. Elson C, Underbakke G, Hanson P, Shrago E, et al.

Int J Crude Drug Res. 1989;27 (2) 121-126 Evaluation of the antifungalactivity of Lemongrass Oil. Onawunmi G O.

The Energetics of Western Herbs Holmes, P., Natrop Publishing. 1989

Journal of Laboratory and Clinical Medicine 1988 Feb;111(2):224-8 Blood coagulation in postmenopausal women given estrogen treatment: comparison of transdermal and oral administration. Alkjaersig N, Fletcher AP, de Ziegler D, Steingold KA, Meldrum DR, Judd HL.

Medico Biologic Information. 1988 3: 8-14 Rose oil: acute and subacute oral toxicity. Kirow M, Bainova A, Spasovski M.

Medico Biologic Information. 1988 3: 18-22.18-22 Rose oil: Lipotropic effect in modeled fatty dystrophy of the liver. Kirow M, Burkova et al.

Indian Pediatrics, Vol 24, Issue 12 12/87 1111-6 Oil Application in Preterm Babies- A Source Of Warmth and Nutrition. Fernandez, A., Patkar, S. et al.

Microbios. 1987 50: 43-59 Effects of lemongrass oil on the morphological characteristics andpeptidoglycan synthesis of Escherichia coli cells. Ogunlana E O, Hoglund S, Onawunmi G O, Skold O.

American Heart Journal 1986 Jul;112(1):229-32 Some issues concerning transdermal nitroglycerin patches. Atkins JM.

Int J Crude Drug Research. 1986 24(2) 64-68. A Study of theantibacterial activity of the EO of Lemongrass. Onawunmi G & Ogunlana E.

Journal of Clinical Endocrinology and Metabolism 1985 Oct;61(4):627-32 Treatment of hot flashes with transdermal estradiol administration. Steingold KA, Laufer L, Chetkowski RJ, DeFazio JD, Matt DW, Meldrum DR, Judd HL.

Pharmacological Research Communications 1985 Jun;17(6):501-12 Skin penetration of minerals in psoriatics and guinea-pigs bathing in hypertonic salt solutions. Shani J, Barak S, Levi D, Ram M, Schachner ER, Schlesinger T, Robberecht H, Van Grieken R, Avrach WW.

Am. J. of Public Health 1984; 74(5):479-84 The Role of Skin Absorption as a Route of Exposure for Volatile Organic Compounds (VOC's) in Drinking Water. Brown, H.S., Bishop, DR., Rowan, CA.

A Modern Herbal Grieve M., London: Penguin 1984, p. 627

Arzneimittelforschung 1982;32(1):56-8 (Published in German) [Percutaneous absorption of various terpenes -menthol, camphene, limonene, isoborneol-acetate, alpha-pinene - from foam baths (author's transl)] Schafer R, Schafer W.

307

Plant Med Phytther 1982 16 (4) 260-279 Contribution to the study on plants used in traditional medicine in Tunisia. Boukef K, Souissi H R, Balansard G.

The Practice of Aromatherapy Valnet J., Rochester, Vermont; Destiny Books, 1980

Fitoterapia 1980 51: 201-205 Antimicrobial activity of some Egyptian aromatic plants. Ross S A, El-Keltawi N E. Megalla S E.

J Ethnopharmacology 2, 1980 4: 337-344 Fennel & Anise as estrogenic agents. Albert-Puleo M.

Bull Med Ethnobot Res. 1980 1: 401-407 Chemical study and antimicrobial properties of essential oil of Cymbopogon citratus. Agarwal I, Kharwal H B, Methela C S.

Journal of Ethnopharmacology. 1979 1: 303-306. Plants in traditional medicine. Marini-Bettolo GB.

American Journal of Clinical Nutrition 1977 Apr;30(4):528-30 Zinc absorption through skin: correction of zinc deficiency in the rat. Keen CL, Hurley LS.

Indian J Expl Biol. 1976 May: 14(3) 370-1 Effect of EO of C citratus on CNS. Seth, Kokate,Varma.

Folia Med. 1969 11 (5) 307-317 The neuro-psychic effect of Bulgarian rose, lavender and geranium. Tasev T, Toleva P, Balabanova V.

Wein Med Wochenschr. 1968 15:345-350 A review of clinical, pharmacological and bacteriological research into Oleum spicae. Von Frohlich E.

Vet Med Nauki 1968 5(6)63-69. Shipochliev T. Pharmacological investigationinto several essential oils: effect on smooth muscles.

Angew Chem Int Ed Engl 1. 1962 537-547 Biology and biochemistry of reproduction and contraception. Jochle W.

Bulletin of MedicalEthnobotony Research. 1960;1, p 401-407 Preliminary phytochemical study of Cymbopogon citratus. Alves A, Pista N & Figeira de Sousa A.

J Agric Food Chem. 39: 660-662 Effects of essential oils on glutathione S-Transferase activi ty in mice. Lam L K, Zheng B.

INDEX

313

ADDITIONAL HEALTH TITLES
FROM HOHM PRESS

■ <u>AFTER SURGERY, ILLNESS OR TRAUMA:</u> *10 Practical Steps to Renewed Energy and Health*
by Regina Sara Ryan   Foreword by John W. Travis, M.D.
This book fills the important need of helping us survive and even thrive through our necessary "down-time" in recuperating from surgery, trauma or illness. Learn a wellness-approach to recuperation that addresses: how to manage and reduce pain; coping with fear, anger, frustration and other unexpected emotions; keeping inspired for renewed life, during and after recovery; becoming an active participant in your own healing; how to deal with well-meaning visitors and caregivers...and more.
Paper, 240 pages, $14.95   ISBN: 0-934252-95-5

■ <u>A VEGETARIAN DOCTOR SPEAKS OUT</u>
by Charles Attwood, M.D., F.A.A.P.
By the famed author of *Dr. Attwood's Low-Fat Prescription for Kids* (Viking, 1995), this new book proclaims the life-saving benefits of a plant-based diet. Twenty-six powerful essays speak out against the myths, the prejudices and the ignorance surrounding the subject of nutrition in the U.S. today. Read about the link between high-fat consumption and heart disease, cancer and other killers; the natural and non-dairy way to increase calcium intake; obesity and our children—more than a matter of genes!; controlling food allergies, for the rest of your life, and many more topics of interest and necessity.
Paper, 216 pages, $14.95   ISBN: 0-934252-85-8

■ <u>10 ESSENTIAL FOODS</u>
by Lalitha Thomas
Presents 10 ordinary but *essential* and great-tasting foods that can: • Strengthen a weakened immune system • Rebalance brain chemistry • Fight cancer and other degenerative diseases • Help you lose weight, simply and naturally. Carrots, broccoli, almonds, grapefruit and six other miracle foods will enhance your health when used regularly and wisely. Each chapter contains easy and delicious recipes, tips for feeding kids and helpful hints for managing your food dollar. A bonus section supports the use of 10 Essential Snacks.
Paper, 324 pages, $16.95   ISBN: 0-934252-74-2

■ <u>10 ESSENTIAL HERBS, REVISED EDITION</u>
by Lalitha Thomas
Peppermint...Garlic...Ginger...Cayenne...Clove...and 5 other everyday herbs win the author's vote as the "Top 10" most versatile and effective herbal applications for hundreds of health and beauty needs. *Ten Essential Herbs* offers fascinating stories and easy, step-by-step direction for both beginners and seasoned herbalists. Special sections in each chapter explain the application of these herbs with children and pets too.
Paper, 396 pages, $16.95   ISBN: 0-934252-48-3

- **NATURAL HEALING WITH HERBS**
by Humbart Santillo, N.D.   Foreword by Robert S. Mendelsohn, M.D.
Acclaimed as the most comprehensive work of its kind, this book details
in simple terms the properties and uses of 120 of the most common herbs
and lists comprehensive therapies for more than 140 common ailments.
Includes special sections on: • Diagnosis • How to make herbal remedies
• The nature of health and disease • Diet and detoxification •
Homeopathy. . .and more. Over 175,000 copies in print.
Paper, 408 pages, $16.95   ISBN: 0-934252-08-4

- **FOOD ENZYMES:** *The Missing Link to Radiant Health*
by Humbart "Smokey" Santillo, N.D.
This book explains how the body's immune system, as well as every
other human metabolic function, requires enzymes in order to work
properly. Dr. Santillo's breakthrough book presents the most current
research in this field and encourages simple, straightforward steps for
how to make enzyme supplementation a natural addition to a nutrition-
conscious lifestyle. Special sections on: • Longevity and disease • The
value of raw food and juicing • Detoxification • Prevention of allergies
and candida • Sports and nutrition.
Over 200,000 copies in print.
Paper, 108 pages, U.S. $7.95, ISBN: 0-934252-40-8 (English)
Now available in Spanish language version.
Paper, 108 pages, U.S. $6.95, ISBN: 0-934252-49-1 (Spanish)

- **INTUITIVE EATING:** *Everybody's Natural Guide to Total Health
and Lifelong Vitality Through Food*
by Humbart "Smokey" Santillo, N.D.
This book details the basics of nutrition and helps the reader to transition
from a toxic diet to a natural, healthy diet. *Intuitive Eating* offers tested
methods for: • strengthening the immune system • natural weight loss
• increasing energy • slowing the aging process. Includes meal plans,
recipes and charts of the nutritional content of most common foods.
Paper, 444 pages, $16.95   ISBN: 0-934252-27-0

- **YOUR BODY CAN TALK:** *How to Use Simple Muscle Testing to
Learn What Your Body Knows and Needs*
by Susan L. Levy, D.C. and Carol Lehr, M.A.
This elegant manual on clinical kinesiology contains a simple method of
energetic muscle testing to help you decode symptoms of body
dysfunction. • Discover your food sensitivities • Determine effects of
electromagnetic pollution in your home or workplace • Evaluate the
strength of your heart, your kidneys, your liver • Test your immune
system functioning • Choose which treatment methods will best handle
your condition. Special Chapters for Women cover issues of PMS and
Menopause. Special Chapter for Men deals with stress and heart disease,
impotence and prostate problems.
Paper, 390 pages, $19.95   ISBN: 0-934252-68-8

■ **MANAGING AND PREVENTING PROSTATE DISORDERS:**
The Natural Alternatives
by George L. Redmon, Ph.D., N.D.
Lifesaving information every man should know about, who is at risk, prevention options and safe natural treatments for prostate disorders. Includes a twenty-five step wellness plan, a personalized maintenance program, and a complete resource and referral guide. Dr. Redmon shows how mind, body and emotions interact with and promote the overall health of the immune system. Prevention and treatment options feature: nutritional recommendations, enzyme therapies, herbs and supplements, detoxification programs, and much more.
Paper, 185 pages, $12.95 ISBN 0-934252-97-91

■ **GINGER: COMMON SPICE & WONDER DRUG**
by Paul Schulick
(published by Herbal Free Press, Brattleboro, Vermont)
A growing classic in the field of herbal medicine, Paul Schulick's first book links the claims of ancient herbalists about the remarkable healing power of ginger to the extensive findings of modern day international medical research. Supported by hundreds of scientific references, this book leads the reader through ginger's 5000-year history to discover the extraordinary and personal benefits of using this miracle herb today.
"A wonderful collection of information. A convincing case."—Andrew Weil, M.D.
Paper, 176 pages, $9.95 ISBN: 0-9639297-1-2

■ **BEYOND ASPIRIN**:
Nature's Answer To Arthritis, Cancer & Alzheimer's Disease
by Thomas A. Newmark and Paul Schulick
A reader-friendly guide to one of the most remarkable medical breakthroughs of our times. Research shows that inhibition of the COX-2 enzyme significantly reduces the inflammation that is currently linked with arthritis, colon and other cancers, and Alzheimer's disease. Challenging the conventional pharmaceutical "silver-bullet" approach this book pleads a convincing case for the safe and effective use of the COX-2-inhibiting herbs, including green tea, rosemary, basil, ginger, turmeric and others.
Paper, 340 pages, $14.95 ISBN: 0-934252-82-3

AUDIO CASSETTES BY
HUMBART "SMOKEY" SANTILLO, N.D.

■ **HERBS, NUTRITION AND HEALING**
Santillo's most comprehensive seminar series. Topics covered in-depth include: • the history of herbology • specific preparation of herbs for tinctures, salves, concentrates, etc. • herbal dosages in both acute and chronic illnesses • use of cleansing and transition diets • treating colds and flu. 4 cassettes, 330 minutes, $40.00, ISBN: 0-934252-22-X

■ **NATURE HEALS FROM WITHIN**
How to take the next step in improving your life and health through nutrition. Topics include: • The innate wisdom of the body • The essential role of elimination and detoxification • Improving digestion • How "transition dieting" will take off the weight—for good! • The role of heredity, diet, and prevention in health • How to overcome tiredness, improve your immune system and live longer...and happier.
1 cassette, $8.95, ISBN: 0-934252-66-1

■ **FOOD ENZYMES:** *Live Educational Seminar*
An in-depth discussion of the properties of food enzymes, describing their valuable use to maintain vitality, immunity, health and longevity. A must for anyone interested in optimal health. Complements all the information in the book. 1 cassette, $8.95, ISBN: 0-934252-29-7

■ **FOOD ENZYMES:** *The Missing Link to Radiant Health*
The audio book form of our bestselling health book. Makes learning easy and interesting. Read by author and radio personality Steve Ball.
2 cassettes, $17.95, ISBN: 0-934252-11-4

■ **FRUITS AND VEGETABLES:** *The Basis of Health*
Juicing of fruits and vegetables is one of the fastest and most efficient ways to supply the body with the raw food nutrients and enzymes needed to maintain optimal health. Explains the essential difference between a live food diet, which heals the body, and degenerative foods, which weaken the immune system and cause disease. Recipes included.
1 cassette, $8.95, ISBN: 0-934252-65-3

■ **WEIGHT-LOSS SEMINAR**
"The healthiest people in the world know the secret of weight loss," says Santillo in this candid, practical, and information-based seminar. This seminar explains the worthlessness of most dietary regimens and explodes many common myths about weight gain. Covers: • The essential distinction between "good" fats and "bad" fats • The necessity for protein and how to use it efficiently • How to get primary vitamins and minerals from food • How to ease into becoming an "intuitive eater."
1 cassette, $8.95, ISBN: 0-934252-75-0

RETAIL ORDER FORM FOR HOHM PRESS BOOKS

NAME _____

ADDRESS _____

CITY _____ STATE _____

ZIP _____

QTY	TITLE	ITEM PRICE	TOTAL PRICE
	BOOKS		
_____	BEYOND ASPIRIN-PAPERBACK	$14.95	_____
_____	BEYOND ASPIRIN-HARDCOVER	$24.95	_____
_____	GINGER: COMMON SPICE & WONDER DRUG	$ 9.95	_____
_____	AFTER SURGERY, ILLNESS OR TRAUMA	$14.95	_____
_____	A VEGETARIAN DOCTOR SPEAKS OUT	$14.95	_____
_____	10 ESSENTIAL FOODS	$16.95	_____
_____	10 ESSENTIAL HERBS, REVISED EDITION	$16.95	_____
_____	NATURAL HEALING WITH HERBS	$16.95	_____
_____	FOOD ENZYMES	$ 7.95	_____
_____	FOOD ENZYMES (SPANISH)	$ 6.95	_____
_____	INTUITIVE EATING	$16.95	_____
_____	YOUR BODY CAN TALK	$19.95	_____
_____	MANAGING . . . PROSTATE DISORDERS	$12.95	_____
	AUDIO CASSETTES		
_____	HERBS, NUTRITION AND HEALING	$40.00	_____
_____	NATURE HEALS FROM WITHIN	$ 8.95	_____
_____	FOOD ENZYMES: *Live Educational Seminar*	$ 8.95	_____
_____	FOOD ENZYMES: *The Missing Link to Radiant Health*	$17.95	_____
_____	FRUITS AND VEGETABLES: *The Basis of Health*	$ 8.95	_____
_____	WEIGHT-LOSS SEMINAR	$ 8.95	_____

SUBTOTAL	
SHIPPING	
TOTAL	

SURFACE SHIPPING CHARGES
1st book $4.00
Each additional item $1.00
SHIP MY ORDER
☐ Surface U.S. Mail—Priority ☐ UPS (Mail + $2.00)
☐ 2nd-Day Air (Mail + $5.00) ☐ Next-Day Air (Mail + $15.00)
METHOD OF PAYMENT:
☐ Check or M.O. Payable to Hohm Press, P.O. Box 2501, Prescott, AZ 86302
☐ Call 1-800-381-2700 to place your credit card order
☐ Or call 1-520-717-1779 to fax your credit card order
☐ Information for Visa/MasterCard order only:
Card #_____ – _____ – _____ – _____
Expiration Date _____

Visit our Website to view our complete catalog: www.hohmpress.com
ORDER NOW! Call 1-800-381-2700 or fax your order to 1-520-717-1779.

ABOUT THE AUTHORS

Thomas M. Newmark held a distinguished practice as a civil litigator for almost twenty years. His clients ranged from multinational corporations to environmental defense leagues. In 1996, he served as lead counsel for two major political third parties in their bid for inclusion in the presidential debates.

Tom now devotes his full time to research and writing on herbal medicine. A brilliant and entertaining speaker and educator, he is a frequent guest on both radio and TV, and lectures widely on behalf of the healing power of botanicals. Tom, his wife Terry, and their five children, live in St. Louis, Missouri and Fairfield, Iowa. Terry illustrated the herbs for this book.

Paul Schulick is the author of the bestselling book, *Ginger: Common Spice & Wonder Drug*, now in its third edition. A respected researcher, lecturer and formulator of natural therapeutic products, Paul received certification as a master herbalist from the renowned Dr. John Christopher.

Paul currently focuses on international scientific research in herbal medicine, exploring The National Library of Medicine, Napralert, Medline, Biosis and Agricola. Rooted in traditional herbalism, Paul utilizes database research to rigorously substantiate herbalism's time-honored claims. He lives and works in Brattleboro, Vermont with his wife Barbi and their children, Geremy and Rosalie, just down the road from Rudyard Kipling's home in the Black Mountains.

HOHM PRESS publishes works in the fields of health, personal transformation, poetry, fine spiritual literature and children's books. If this book was of interest to you, we will be happy to send you a catalog.

Name _____

Street or box number _____

City _____

State _____ Zip _____

☐ PLEASE DO NOT PUT MY NAME ON YOUR MAILING LIST.

HOHM PRESS
P.O. Box 2501
Prescott, Arizona 86302